The
Million
Dollar Code

When Healthcare Hurts Instead of Heals
The journey from a healthy athlete to a
medical nightmare.

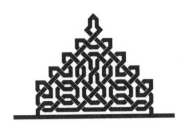

BEN DALES AND B. B. BEAUDREAUX

ISBN: i978-0-578-61415-1

Beaudreaux Publications

P. O. Box 955

Douglas, MI 49406

www.medicaldevicestory.com

Ordering Information:

Bulk Orders: Special discounts are available on quantity purchases by corporations, associations, and others. For details, contact the publisher at the address above.

Table of Contents

Ben Dales and B. B. Beaudreaux

A Note from the Authors

There comes a time in each of our lives when we can choose to do something or choose to do nothing.

Who is to take the first step? Do I? Or is that best left to someone else?

This book project is a result of the latter of these questions. A decision had to be made. A story had to be told. Had the experience not unfolded as it did and twisted every aspect of the lives of those affected, the story may well have remained untold. It may have passed over into oblivion, a story that dies when the involved characters die.

Yet, this is a story that has come to fruition. It was time, and yes, my time to speak up.

Although this story is primarily about the life of two people, it represents so much more. It has repercussions for many who are facing or have faced any medical challenge. It has repercussions for the many who are closely affected by those with these challenges. Thus, although this story is in many ways a tragedy, it would be a far bigger tragedy not to tell it at all.

Ben Dales and B. B. Beaudreaux

We talk in life about the degrees of separation between and among us. If we are closely connected, the choice we make becomes quite clear to help. It is less clear when there a single degree of separation. The choice becomes muddled if there is more separation.

This book contains both a heartwarming story and also a heartbreaking story. The story is simply a result of a decision not to sit by idly while letting someone else (hopefully) help. Those of us who have involved ourselves in this book project are persons who have at long last decided that enough is enough. It is time to stand up. It is time to help.

Consider this quote from a Hindu teaching:

There are hundreds of paths up the mountain, all leading in the same direction, so it doesn't matter which path you take. The only one wasting time is the one who runs around and around the mountain, telling everyone that his or her path is wrong.

The point is that all paths lead to the same peak. We wish for you a journey to the summit filled with intrigue, understanding, compassion, and empathy. We hope you are able to see the forest and not just the trees. Be brave, stoic, and honest with yourself. Most of all, live your life with dignity and grace so that in the end, you will know you fulfilled your destiny with integrity.

The End

Existence or death?

How many of us have pondered this question?

Terminally ill people face this question when their hour is getting near. Do they hang on to every last breath in quiet contemplation and acceptance, or are they so afraid of what awaits them, they go kicking and screaming all the way?

Would you choose to suffer continued horrible pain so that you might live a little longer?

I have often thought that people who die suddenly of a heart attack are so very lucky. They never have to ask themselves questions like these.

Traveling to Belgium was a grueling trip in itself. I knew it would be. I didn't tell Deni, my

spouse and caregiver, where I was going or why. What other option did I have? It was

not that I wanted to keep things shrouded in mystery or to hush things up. No, that was

not it at all. It was just was just that ending my life in the same house we had shared would only bring back horrible memories of that final day to all who stepped foot in our home--as

welcoming and loving and comfortable as it was. I couldn't do that to Deni.

I endured decades of suffering because the pain medications prescribed to me were not strong enough to control the chronic pain.

There was no joy in life--just endless suffering. I couldn't handle it anymore.

I contacted Franny, a widow from Brussels. Franny's husband, Jens, had brain cancer and chose to leave this world while he still had the mental capacity to know whom he still loved. He made this choice in order to avoid all the harrowing drama that brain cancer causes as tumors increase in size, taking away all the personality the victim has, while suffering a prolonged death. His choice made absolute sense to him, even if not for her. She, being a physician, had seen death, but watching her husband decline was a different story. Franny had told me all about the ordeal, how unforgettably draining it was for her. This is why I had to keep this last episode from Deni.

I didn't want the one I loved to watch me die. Deni would have been too emotional. It would have been too much for both of us.

Ben Dales and B. B. Beaudreaux

Franny and Jens got to say their last goodbyes and embrace in each other's arms as the fatal dosage of chemicals were administered through the IV (intravenous apparatus) within the familiar setting of their own home in Brussels. Belgium was one of the first countries in the world to legalize physician-assisted euthanasia for humans. For them, it was the most compassionate act to take for the love of one's life.

I had met Franny on a social media website where she was speaking about the positive transition period of her husband and why she was an advocate for self-euthanasia. For her, the suffering she already saw her loved one go through was painful enough without having to watch him go mad as the tumor grew.

Franny related to me how a young woman on the west coast of the United States had the same dilemma as Jens and was carrying around a lethal combination of drugs. She carried the drugs just in case it got to the point of such suffering that she would have the means necessary to end her life, even if the pills were a painful way to go. She and her husband had to move to Oregon, where she could legally be prescribed this dual dosage of drugs to complete this final act of compassion.

As for me, I suppose I could still derive enjoyment out of continuing to stay alive, but the truth was, the morphine had become more and more ineffective, making it difficult to hide my pain in my daily life.

Ending my life a world away seemed to be the right thing to do. I didn't want my loved ones to see me at my final moments.

The anesthesiologist who helped Franny's husband and would be helping me, Dr. Rand, had consulted with me previously. He told me I had to be one-hundred percent sure that I wanted to go through with this procedure. Fran was letting me stay at her home, which was a modernly-renovated apartment in what most of us would call a row house. Row house streets were plentiful in Brussels and very attractive as well, with each exterior of a different color as one walked down the street. Franny knew, by offering her home, that she was helping me with the most difficult decision anyone could ever face.

Dr. Rand had already initiated me into the entire procedure twice before during this trip, both times in Franny's living room area. Amidst the modern motif of this room, there were many touches which made me feel like I was in "Old Europe." Ornate picture frames surrounded what looked like many family photos. The atmosphere, if not smell, of the room gave hints of dried spices and herbs. Large windows emitted filtered light through paper-like blinds from the second story view of a small

Ben Dales and B. B. Beaudreaux

park across the street. Typically, Fran would be enjoying background classical music through the small speakers mounted on the walls.

In each of the two previous tries at this, an IV had been hooked up to my arm while I was lying comfortably on the modern yet comfortable deep blue fabric sofa. Just Dr. Rand, Franny, and her dog Max were there with me on each occasion. Max was a Malinois, or more commonly known as a Belgian shepherd. Though a bit smaller, he reminded me of one of my best pets ever--my German shepherd Heidi, who had given me fifteen wonderful years as my service dog.

In any case, I indeed was now feeling like a dog one brings to the vet to have put to sleep.

Twice, in the past few days, I chickened out. I just could not end my life.

Dr. Rand reminded me that I did not have to go through with anything and that he was willing to treat me here in Brussels for the rest of my life. He could prescribe as much medication as I needed, and I could go on having some semblance of a life--as difficult as it was. He told me that it was his job to ease people's suffering. He saw this compassionate mission as a way for him to lead his life. It was his hope that there would be someone to help him as need be at life's end, just as he had been helping others in this same way. This was just the very reason why I wanted him here now.

I didn't want to suffer anymore.

Two times before, we had set up the IV and prepared what would be necessary to administer a sedative in preparation for the end. Dr. Rand proceeded to have the final conversation with me in order to ensure I was ready. In both instances, I became too anxious, my nerves getting the best of me, and so the IV was removed and things packed up to wait for the time I felt was appropriate.

Dr. Rand assured me, "I will set up a million times if need be, Ted. Only you can make the ultimate decision."

"But I'm running out of money."

"Ted, the money doesn't matter to me. I will do this a million times, and I will stop it a million times if it doesn't feel right to you."

I thought about how taxing this had to be for Fran, but there was no anxiety coming my way from her. All Fran wanted to do was help me. I was so very lucky to have found her.

I told Franny that it was she who would have to write what happened at the end, since I was going to die and would not be able to finish the last

Ben Dales and B. B. Beaudreaux

chapter in my medical journal. I had already signed my cadaver over to medical science in Belgium in order to reveal and document what brought me to choose to end my life during the decade that was supposed to have been the prime of my life.

Franny also agreed to inform Deni what happened and to offer to help my spouse as much as possible.

This was the third time the doctor had set up the IV and the medications that would end my life. I was thinking I could not have him keep doing this--I had to decide that this was truly the end.

As the sedative was administered once again, I was fighting and I was nervous. I started crying.

I thought about all the things I had not accomplished. I thought about all the dreams that I once had that would never happen.

I was once a very active athlete with a full life. A series of medical mistakes took away all of those dreams.

I recalled the old adage: when accountants make mistakes, they use an eraser and fix it. But doctors? Doctors bury their mistakes.

By now, I was crying and extremely upset. I was angry with the medical profession. I was angry with the insurance industry, the cause of all the botched medical procedures that happened to me. I was angry with the medical device industry. The unfinished story about how this all happened to me, going from a healthy athlete to being crippled by daily pain, was overwhelming.

I wished I never even had medical insurance at all. Yet, it had been pounded into my head since I was a kid, "Oh, don't ever be without insurance--you could lose everything if you have an accident." At least, this is how people in the United States were conditioned to think.

Truth be told, I lost my healthy life because I had medical insurance. Maybe my life would have had a different ending if I hadn't gone on the insurance-driven medical merry-go-round. The medical field had changed so very much since I was a child. It was no longer about caring for people. It was almost exclusively about making money for the founders, the stockholders, and the corporate executives.

And now it was literally killing me.

I started flailing and pulled out one of the IV tubes, blood spilling on the floor.

Dr. Rand immediately clapped off the tube and reinserted it to the IV drip hanging behind my head.

Ben Dales and B. B. Beaudreaux

I was babbling now. I was agitated. I was furious.

Fran and the doctor were speaking in their native French, some of which I could understand. I was thinking they were saying, "Let's just end his suffering."

I was screaming, "FINE! FINE! Just kill me NOW!"

"You are not in the right frame of mind, Ted. And...I have never killed a patient. This is not how it's supposed to end," Dr. Rand replied with a heavy French accent.

"Just kill me now! I'm out of money! I can't stand the constant pain anymore. Just do it now!" I started shaking.

"You are too agitated," Dr. Rand said. "You cannot continue like this. You will have a stroke. Is that how you wish to die?"

"Then just end it! Do it NOW!"

The doctor pulled out a large syringe. This was the end. I was convulsing and crying. I urinated in my pants, but had the forethought to have on an adult diaper. The room started spinning, spinning.

I thought back to my life.

My career. The volleyball games. The skiing. The trips. My friends. All the wonderful meals.

And Deni.

How could I leave this world without Deni?

"Franny, where are you?"

"I'm here," I heard her say. I felt her hand on mine. This was it. This was how I was going to die. Franny was going to be the last person on earth to touch me.

Deni. I wish Deni was here.

I tried to scream, but I could only whimper. "Give Deni all my love."

"I will," Franny replied.

The spinning room was now getting darker, though the sun had been shining when we set up.

Darker still, now black.

My God, how could it have come to this?

Nothingness...

CHAPTER 1

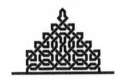

Ted: The Beginning

I was born in 1964, when the emphasis on health was part of the Kennedy administration and thus was the "law of the land"--or at least, of the public schools. For me, from the first grade all the way through high school, physical education was mandatory for all students. This was combined with an emphasis on health education which, at least in the public schools, encompassed learning priorities on hygiene and all that young people might do to be well accepted by their peers and others. Therefore, it became a given that personal hygiene, diet, and exercise were fundamental parts of each student's daily routine.

And so the die was cast for me.

As a child I was extremely nimble. My parents and grandparents were always consistently amazed by the physical feats and activities I was able to achieve on my own. Whether it was climbing trees, riding bicycles or just running or swimming, there was never any fear among my adult supervisors that I would somehow get injured. Of course, I endured the usual scraped knees and the bumps on the head that naturally accompany growth and interaction with others, but for me, my physical agility somehow never led me into any situation where I needed medical attention. I never had a broken bone or even a wound needing stitches. My propensity to become physically injured was practically nil.

Admittedly I did not have the encouragement of my parents to engage in organized sports activities, as they were too wrapped up in their own problems of adult life to bother with me. Even so, I always found myself working hard to further my physical agility and stamina. At first, tumbling was what I loved. I found that by utilizing forward motion, I could make--literally--leaps and bounds through space. It was easy for me and many of my friends compared my agility to that of a cat. I always landed on my feet.

Swimming and cycling were easy and enjoyable; however, those activities required the utilization of outside items, namely a bicycle or a swimming pool. Being a relatively poor kid, these activities were less accessible to me. Bicycling became less prohibitive when I entered my teenage years. Being clever, I could always find old bikes and parts that the wealthier people in suburban areas would put out on the curb for the trash. I hunted for discarded bicycles and parts in the afternoons and evenings before next-day garbage pickup. I began to build and fashion my own bicycles.

Swimming likewise turned out to be a non-issue, because scaling the fenced wall of the community pool after nightfall was a most easy thing for me as a climber to do. The pool had a diving board of nine and three meters. As far as heights like that were concerned, I had absolutely no fear whatsoever.

My childhood was not just about sports and physical agility, however. In fourth grade, I took a musical aptitude test. This revealed a potential hidden talent, as I achieved the highest score among our school's fourth-graders. The director of the music program recruited me into learning to play the cello. Additional testing revealed I had what was known as perfect vocal pitch. I joined the choral program as well.

Moving onto middle school and then high school, I became disenfranchised from the more affluent kids whose parents lived their own unaccomplished dreams vicariously by forcing their children into sports and musical activities that they wished they had participated in as children. My parents never pushed me into anything. In fact, it was because of the divorce of my parents, along with what can be labeled as just an absolute lack of involvement in my life, which led me to seek out sports and music on my own.

There was one other major life happening that absolutely changed everything. My father nearly died in an automobile accident when I was in sixth grade. He actually had been declared D.O.A. (Dead On Arrival) at the hospital due to massive brain and head injuries. He was lucky— he regained consciousness and lived. However, he was never the same after the accident; he lost mental capacities as a result. This took away his ability to maintain meaningful employment and provide for his four children.

What this meant for me was an end to my participation in sports and other school activities, including music. Instead I found odd jobs in order to have food to eat and clothes to wear. This situation took a toll on my school attendance, which affected my grades. I ended up in summer school just to keep up with my classmates.

I never told anyone at school what had actually transpired with my dad. I knew that revealing what was going on at home would reflect on my parents, meaning school officials would likely have tried to interfere with my home life. I just did whatever I could to appear normal and to make up for class time missed as a result of having to work. I found myself preemptively signing up for difficult mandatory courses such as U.S. History during the summer of my freshman year of high school instead of waiting until the usual junior year. In this way I was able to complete a year-long course in a little over five weeks.

If there was any benefit to my need to work, it was that getting back and forth to the many odd jobs and temporary work was always by bicycle. My legs became very powerful, as I truly enjoyed the sport of cycling even if for work purposes.

Little did I know that I would one day look back, and wish I could ride a bicycle again.

CHAPTER 2

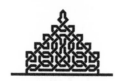

Deni: Meeting On The "El"

I met Ted on the "El" (Elevated Trains) in Chicago, where we were both daily commuters.

It was common for me to see some of the same faces repeatedly during my daily commutes. Usually I never really spoke to or met the people behind those faces.

This time it was different. I distinctly recall being on opposite ends of the same train car, both of us standing as ample seating for all is never the case during rush hours. We caught each other's eyes somehow and continued our mutual gazing. Some would simply call this the act of flirting. In any case, we continued to hold each other's eyes again and again throughout the twenty-minute ride downtown. We ended it with a slight but inviting smile. He was the one who had to break it when he departed the train at his usual downtown stop-

-two stops before mine. It was an incredible first meeting, even if no words were exchanged. Here was an incredibly handsome man, impeccably dressed in a dark suit, white shirt and tie, who seemed to be interested in me.

When I arrived at my office, I told a close work friend, "I think I just saw the love of my life on the train."

During the next two months or so, the two of us repeated our nonverbal encounters on the train perhaps three or four more times. There was no chance for any verbal communication during these commutes with the trains so full. We were not on the same train repeatedly throughout these months. There are eight cars per train with the various trains going downtown coming about every fifteen minutes. Thus, it is possible, even likely, to be on a different train any given day if one is running late or if the trains are behind schedule. The odds of being in the very same car on the same train at the same time are slim. All I knew for sure about him is that he certainly had a professional position downtown, as each time I encountered him, he was dressed in the most professional attire.

One morning I entered another typically full train and proceeded to one end of the car, as the loudspeaker recorded announcements always direct everyone to do. There he was, in a window seat near the car's end, just two seats away from where I stood. He was reading the morning *Chicago Tribune* and did not see me.

At the very first stop after I boarded, the seat just adjacent to his was vacated by a woman in medical scrubs. I quickly moved over to replace the woman sitting next to him.

"Hi."

He turned to look at me.

"Hi, I'm Ted."

"I'm Deni. I've seen you a couple of times."

This led to enough other conversation to strike a chord of familiarity, if not attraction. I gave him my business card before his stop and asked him to feel free to call me for lunch sometime.

I did not see him the next couple of times on the train. He didn't call me about having lunch. Though I was a bit disappointed, I simply chalked it up to happenstance and did not dwell on it. However, I have to admit I was more than just a bit curious about what professional position he held and about the personality behind that inviting smile.

The day came again a few weeks later when it happened all over again, a chance to talk some

Ben Dales and B. B. Beaudreaux

more on the morning train. This time more definite plans were made, and we met for lunch at one of the Loop restaurants in the underground Pedway. During this lunch, as fun and even romantic as it was, we both admitted we normally did not "go out for lunch" but instead brought our own homemade lunches from home. With this in common, we decided to bring our respective home lunches outside to eat together on one of the benches in the wonderfully landscaped gardens of the Art Institute of Chicago, as it was summer weather then.

Lunches from home became a habit and turned into a picnic as each of us would plan to bring different food items to share. We both already knew that our own home-prepared lunches were far better and healthier than any fast food establishment in downtown Chicago. The gardens were beautiful and so was the company. Our lunch meetings were lighthearted and fun, as we both were in a "try to impress" mode as we mutually tried to show off culinary talents. When the weather turned colder, we continued to meet for our picnic lunches inside. We found a spacious and comfortable meeting spot in the main lobby of the Chicago Cultural Center, a room filled with lunchtime tables for the public. We continued meeting all winter long until we were able to do so again outside in the welcome warmer spring weather. Whether we lunched inside or outside, our romance continued to grow.

We introduced our lives to each other. I learned he was with the IT department of the largest law firm in the world, while he learned of my airline background leading to my lead trainer position for a large corporate travel management company. I did not realize, though, the importance of his position until he began bringing me for visits to his office. He was actually a top executive for his firm. Following one of these office visits, he surprised me by taking me to dinner at the exclusive Plaza Club at the top of the Prudential Building (just one floor above his office). To this day, I do not believe I have ever been treated more like royalty while dining. I later learned that he was only one of two Plaza Club members from the Executive Floor of the firm; the other was the firm's CEO. Later on, I would learn this was actually a Chicago Society of Clubs membership that gave us access to other partner clubs around the world (one which hosted us for an entire week of pampering at a partner resort in Puerto Rico). I felt appreciated like never before when he treated me to such extravagance.

By this time, we also met each other for other occasions. You might say we had begun dating. The most special part of how all this happened is that we took the time to get to know each other

Ben Dales and B. B. Beaudreaux

and did it just one step at a time. We became friends long before we became lovers. That made the latter happening all the more special when the time came.

We eventually brought each other into our respective circles of friends. Our friends in both circles began kidding us about "becoming an item." We both learned to counter these accusations with wry smiles and correct them by stating, "No, we're just dating." Of course, this went on for months into years. "No, we're just dating!"

After the ease of introductions and acceptances into our circles of friends, we decided to take the next, usual, nerve-racking step of bringing each other into our mutual family circles.

I met his dad first. Ted tried hard to "prepare me" for this meeting. He expressed I should not have high expectations, because as he said his dad was just a simple, not particularly professional man. Ted drove me to his dad's small and simple upstairs apartment in a two-flat building on the far southwest side of Chicago. We pulled up to a two-story brick building on the corner of Kedzie Avenue, a busy street. We entered the building through a side door and climbed up the stairs to the second floor.

The flat was not fancy, nor was it shabby--just kind of "middle of the road." We entered without knocking and walked into the apartment's kitchen. It was modestly set up, and looked as clean as one would expect a bachelor apartment to be (not really clean but not really dirty either). His dad came out of another room to meet and greet me with a smile. He could not have been more friendly and accepting. He talked to me as if he had known me forever. I learned later, delightedly so, that this is how his dad was with everybody. Afterwards, I told Ted that his request for me to have "lowered expectations" was really unnecessary, because I liked his dad just as he was.

I have to say that meeting his mom was even better. Ted drove me to the south suburban home where he had grown up. It was on a quiet, somewhat secluded street with minimal traffic. It was a split-level home, kind of a faded yellow color and quite modest in appearance and size. There was a large apple tree in front that hovered over an old sidewalk leading to the front door. I learned later, he took me through the front door mostly to impress me, as ever since then we have always entered by the side door from the driveway (like all family members do).

His mom was seated on a sectional sofa, with the TV on and avidly reading a book. "Hi, Mom.

Ben Dales and B. B. Beaudreaux

I want you to meet Deni. Deni--this is my mom, LaVerne. Everyone calls her Lovey."

His mom shook my hand. "Hi, I'm Lovey," she said with a smile.

"I love the name LaVerne," I said. "I have three Aunt LaVernes. I'm really close to one of them, my mom's sister."

Ted looked at me in disbelief. "Nobody has three Aunt LaVernes."

"Not only do I have three Aunt LaVernes, but two of them have the same last name since they both married my great-uncles who are brothers of my maternal grandmother."

Ted shot me another look of disbelief. He was sure I was making it all up. He did not know me well enough to know that I'm a terrible liar and can be seen right through when attempting to do so.

I turned to his mom and said, "I will call you LaVerne as it's a favorite name in my family."

"Oh, just call me Mom," she smiled. I thought it was such a kind thing to say.

When we were about to leave and saying our goodbyes, I said, "I'll see you next time, Mom."

As soon as we got into Ted's car, his first words were, "'Just call me Mom'? She wants to keep you in the family, even if I haven't yet made that decision!"

I roared with laughter.

As our relationship developed further (and admittedly, our love), we took trips together. Ted came to Indiana with me to see where I grew up on a corn-and-soybeans farm and to meet some family members. I went with him to his grandparents' old country house in the northwoods of Wisconsin to stay for weekends; sometimes alone with him and sometimes with his family members.

Since my work involved travel benefits, we were able to take some other trips together. Among the various trips we took domestically (in the U.S.) were many that involved Ted's volleyball competitions and tournaments. Ted was on three competitive adult volleyball teams, two that competed in Chicago leagues and one that was a traveling team competing in competitions across North America.

We also took various pleasure trips which had no connection to volleyball. You see, my job position during that phase of my life was in travel. We traveled all across North America, including Canada and Mexico. We were able to travel internationally from Europe to South America to New Zealand and Australia. In so doing, we hiked mountains and climbed pyramids. We skied together. We walked miles in most cities, agreeing it was among the best ways really to experience them.

It is said that one of the best ways to judge compatibility is whether two people can travel together. Both of us passed this unintended test with flying colors in each other's eyes. We shared many of the same interests, but if we did not, it was not a problem. We adapted and adjusted during each trip.

We also discovered traits about each other that served to deepen our loving respect more and more. While driving in a rental car together in Los Angeles, we ventured into Pasadena to see the sights. By this time in our relationship, we discovered that not only did we like exploring the popular areas but we both enjoyed taking the back streets and seeing how real people live.

As we drove that day, we found ourselves in an elegant Pasadena neighborhood with many curving, busy streets and cul-de-sacs. While I was driving, Ted suddenly screamed, "Stop the car!"

I thought I had hit something or was about to. I slammed on the brakes and stopped the car in the middle of a busy street. Ted got out immediately and ran over toward a woman on a corner carrying what I thought was a cane and a couple of bags. I pulled over to the side to watch. Ted slowed down his run to a walk as he approached her and said something. The woman looked frightened and appeared to respond in a negative fashion. Ted continued to converse with her. I watched as this woman visibly relaxed and allowed him to take her arm as if to be escorted. Ted continued to talk to her as he helped her to cross the street at the corner and then walked her to another corner. He directed her to turn down the side street. He spoke briefly just a bit more, and she then continued on her own.

"Let's wait and watch to make sure she's okay," Ted said to me when he returned to the car. "She's blind and was a bit lost while trying to go to a friend's house."

I was near tears at this point, listening to his story of how he cared enough to stop to help someone while vacationing in a strange city himself. How he knew that this woman was not only blind, but in distress and frightened, I couldn't figure out. I didn't understand how he knew enough to help her. Ted couldn't see the front of her face as we were driving past, but somehow, he intuitively

Ben Dales and B. B. Beaudreaux

knew that this older, blind woman was in need of assistance.

I loved him just a bit more so after that.

A similar incident happened on Christmas Eve, only about ten miles from my hometown in Indiana. We arrived mid-afternoon at my brother's home for the family Christmas gathering and planned to leave early due to a predicted snowstorm. We had to get back to Chicago for his family's Christmas at his grandmother's the next day.

After the usual Christmas feeding and the frenzy of unwrapping gifts, we packed up gifts received and food packaged for us to take home.

We got in my car and I started out driving slowly on the two-hour drive back to the city. It was already snowing like crazy with near-blizzard conditions. Only fifteen minutes into our drive, I drove past what looked like a man carrying something along this rather isolated state highway.

"Stop the car!" Ted startled me. "Turn around and go back! That guy is carrying something--it looks like a dog."

"Ted, it's a blizzard out there, we need to get back home. The guy is probably just walking to the next house where he lives."

"I think he needs help!"

I relented, turning the car around slowly on the deserted snowy highway. As it turned out, it was a relatively young man who was in fact carrying his dog. However, he was not headed back to his or any nearby house--he was headed to another Indiana town about an hour away.

The back seat of our car was filled with some large gifts and boxes of food, yet we made room for him at Ted's insistence that we give him a ride with the wet and shivering rather large dog. We learned this man had already traveled some twenty miles but had a ride for the first eighteen miles right up to the last intersecting highway. He had walked the last couple of miles in the blizzard before we came along. I learned surprisingly that his family home was a neighboring one to one of my mom's distant cousins in the next county south, and that home was where he had been coming from on Christmas Eve. He, with his dog along, had no other way to travel than by hitchhiking.

Even though this man's destination town was a bit out of our way heading to Chicago, we nonetheless helped this man on Christmas Eve and felt all the better for it. It would never have happened just like this, except for the kind and

Ben Dales and B. B. Beaudreaux

caring heart of Ted toward others in need. We even shared our Christmas leftovers with that man that evening, and I'm sure with his dog too.

Again, I loved Ted just a bit more so after that Christmas Eve. Through the years, there have been many other such incidents of our helping others. I have learned from Ted that this is now our norm.

Little did we know then how much these times before and after that Christmas were to be our so-called glory days. We were both healthy and agile enough to do what we felt like doing and our bodies cooperated. His youth helped keep me even more young and agile than I might have been, being some sixteen years and five months older than he.

As I stated earlier, my job involved travel benefits. I ended up winning a free weekend trip that led to our elopement. The prize, won at my travel company's annual summer picnic, was a three-day package at a Vermont ski resort in the picturesque town of Stowe (where the real Von Trapp family of "The Sound of Music" ended up settling). It culminated in our planning an outdoor ceremony in a mountainside gazebo, at high noon on a sunny January day with fresh fallen snow, to which we traversed in a beautifully refurbished sleigh with green velvet seats operated by horse and driver (named Tom and Rochelle respectively). It was just us, except for the local Justice of the Peace, who performed our religious civil ceremony and witnessed our touching and consequently emotional loving exchange of vows.

Life at this point could not have been grander. There was not the slightest inkling of what was to come.

CHAPTER 3

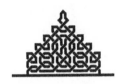

Ted: Power Play

My business trip to the Mexican city of León had been very successful. I upgraded two different systems for two different companies so they would be Y2K-compliant, and did a much-needed hardware upgrade on a facility just north of León that produced FEDEX boxes. This was amidst the beautiful spring weather of Mexico, a much different climate from Chicago. Consequently, making my flights out of León and into Houston for our national volleyball tournament was absolutely not a problem. There had been no required extension of my trip due to various other unexpected computer problems and needs, something not altogether uncommon in my line of work.

Quite frankly, these companies would have been happy to finance my flights to anywhere in the world, considering all the fear instilled in big business about the potentially-apocalyptic Y2K problem. So many people everywhere thought that all the necessary preventive work would never be finished in time by the toll of midnight on December 31, 1999. I knew otherwise. The only thing that was really needed was a database definition change. The computer fields that stored the year stamp of 99 just needed to be increased to include two more digits.

To me, it had been child's play. To the software developers and the hardware producers, it was formally previewed as a two-step process: (a) remove the applicable data from the system, (b) load the new data on the same system with a properly defined database.

A few additional new programs needed to be loaded to handle the two extra digits. In our preparation, we programmers had already run extremely thorough beta tests of every program that could potentially invalidate the time date stamp. To those in the entire tech industry, this was easily the biggest money-making push ever seen in the world of computers.

Design engineers like me knew they held a firm grip in getting a piece of that big golden pie. That is why my trips were paid by my clients. I enjoyed working with my Latin American clients-- maybe because I was able to converse with them in

Ben Dales and B. B. Beaudreaux

Spanish, or maybe it was just the confidence they had in my technical skills. Whatever it was, I felt valued as a competent engineer and a loyal friend that would be there to help them anytime an issue might arise.

However, once the work was completed, I still had my own life to live--and I was going after it! I hopped on a plane to Houston for the North American Volleyball championship tournament.

I loved competitive volleyball, and I was especially excited for this tournament as Deni was meeting me there. Since my team had either won, placed, or showed in at least three different tournaments, we automatically qualified to participate in the North American championship finale. We had done not too shabby of a job throughout the year, so the group we put together was excited about being able to compete in the tournament everyone in the circle viewed as the "culmination" of a year's worth of hard practice and play.

The national volleyball tournament did not go as we had hoped, as our team ended up unexpectedly in third place instead of first. We were the top-seeded team and we expected to win. This is not to say that coming in third in nationals is not respectable; we were just disappointed after the high expectations following preliminaries.

What prevented our winning the championship boiled down to a single play, one which should have been the final point of the match which enigmatically changed on a dime. Yes, and so too was I to learn that one's physical ability, successful career, and even one's incentive to live one's life can change just as quickly.

In the competitive sport of volleyball and its officially-sanctioned tournaments, there are four officials for every game played--two referees and two line judges. The up referee, or "up ref," stands on a ladder or platform at one end of the net and is responsible for the overall management of scoring. His responsibility also includes calls involving a player's going into the net (or even touching it) and for making judgment calls about whether the ball is handled illegally or comes to rest on a player's body.

The down referee, or "down ref," stands on the floor on the opposite end of the net from where the up ref is stationed on the ladder, and his sole responsibility is for calls involving a player's foot going over the solid black line below the net that specifically separates the two teams. This is a very serious and important job as volleyball is a non-contact sport, and having an opponent's foot cross over onto one's own court can lead to a sprained or broken ankle (as actually happened to me before).

The two line judges are positioned in back on opposite corners of the court, and each line judge is responsible for one back boundary line and one side boundary line. In case of any call dispute, it is the up ref who has the final say on the decision.

It was a close game and we were just two points from the win. I had been hitting the ball all around my opponent the entire match, but he was determined to shut me down. Instead of my usual cross-court angled shot, I hit the ball straight down the line in order to catch him off guard.

It worked exactly as I expected, and the ball hit the blocker's hand on the other side of the net. The ball bounced back to our side of the net and then landed **outside** the boundary line on the right side of the court. As the ball hit the floor out of bounds, I looked straight at the line judge positioned at the back corner of the opposing team's court and awaited the obvious call.

His hands immediately went straight up into the air. Out of bounds.

The up ref, also looking at the line judge, blew the whistle and called the point for our team. This call put us at match point. One more point and we would win the entire match and move into the championship.

For some reason, the down ref stopped the game, ran over to the other side of the net where the up ref was on the ladder, and called it "in bounds." This was not even within his jurisdiction to make the call. If anything, it could have been referred to the other line judge, but never to the down ref. In any case, the down ref can never overrule the up ref's call.

To top it all off, the down ref's view was partially blocked by the net pole itself. When we challenged the decision, the up ref ignored the original call of the line judge and backed up the incorrect, unauthorized call made by the down ref. The verbal protests continued, but the up ref appeared to go on some sort of power trip and would not listen--not only to my team but not even to the other team, who also acknowledged the call was wrong.

The fiasco ended up being the turning point for our team in the tournament, as up to now we had been cruising through the winners' bracket. We were unable to pull ourselves out of this terrible call. It was a mental block we just could not shake. We lost that game and the match, and fell into the losers' bracket. We came in third place.

Ben Dales and B. B. Beaudreaux

This was an example of a man who had complete control over the court, would not listen to the truth at all, but only cared about asserting his authority over others and about not admitting such an obvious mistake in both call and ruling.

There is one other curious sidelight to this flashback of the tournament. The down ref, who had overruled the original call with no authority to do so, was actually a volleyball player whom we did not invite to participate with us in the national tournament. We could not help but wonder if his bad call was in retribution.

Looking back at this event years later, I realized the irony of this simple little episode. It was a foreshadowing of how power can corrupt one's judgment. This was just the beginning of one of the most difficult lessons I would learn in life. I would come not only to be hurt by this same type of power corruption in my medical journey but be brought to the end of my life by it.

After the tournament ended, my teammates and I were determined to put it all behind us. I did not let it upset me any further; I was happy just to have been with my friends over the Memorial Day weekend for this tournament.

And now, it was time to celebrate my birthday with Deni. I was so looking forward to this part of the trip even though I had already been traveling for a while. Deni, being a travel agent, had everything set up in advance for the highlight of this journey. I knew the hotel would have us upgraded when Deni set up the reservation for our room using what is known as the "IATA" card (International Air Transport Association). Having one of these cards meant this person was somehow involved in the travel industry, and that always meant upgrading from potential prospects. This made traveling first class so much easier and less expensive than if we had just been any other ordinary couple taking a trip. Plus, Deni was well-known throughout the travel industry--as people tend to talk about who is not only the best in their respective positions in travel, but also one who is, and I quote, "easy on the eyes."

It was at one of the many social functions put on by host hotels that I heard two clients once privately talking in regards to my sweetheart, who would be with me on my birthday weekend. As I recall, the conversation went something like this:

"Hey Chris, that Deni is really something, don't ya think?"

"You mean ya have to 'think' about that?" Chris snickered.

Ben Dales and B. B. Beaudreaux

"And you know what? I heard Deni was a schoolteacher before becoming a trainer for the travel industry," said the first client.

"Well, if I had a teacher like that as a kid," Chris replied, "I would have loved going to class!"

"Who wouldn't have?"

I was lucky to have not only someone good-looking accompanying me, cheering me on. But also a smart, knowledgeable, and well-liked professional setting up all the accommodations for this part of our excursion.

This was definitely going to be one birthday I would never forget!

CHAPTER 4

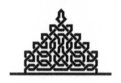

Deni: Birthday Surprise

He related it all to me, after the fact.

Ted told me how in Mexico, the world was his. Once again, it had all gone so well. He had wowed his clients in León, from the top of the company down to the hourly workers. His knowledge and skills had fixed the company's angst over the Y2K computer crisis, even though he was told the problems were insurmountable upon his arrival three days prior. The clients were ready to have him rip out the computers completely and haul them back home to his Chicago company. Of course, I knew that his winning personality and good looks helped turn it all around as well.

As it turned out, he told me they had been so delighted with his work (and with him), he was feted on his final night at the best restaurante in the city, followed by a raucous fiesta in the best cantina in the entire State of León.

Now on his flight departing the dear Mexico he had come to love and respect, Ted shared how he looked out over the picturesque landscape below from seat 2A of his North-bound Mexicana Airlines flight. He toasted his success with his first-class champagne. He told me how it was all so easy, doubly so knowing how he demonstrated his ability and willingness to communicate with his professional amigos in their own idioma.

Ted elected to take Spanish in high school and had not done well. This was attributed in part to his clashes with teachers who were non-native speakers. He was an analytic learner, and far too often his teachers would not answer his many questions of "why" or "what." However, high school Spanish can only go so far. He needed more to make it work in the corporate world of Chicagoland. He recalled the hours spent in perfecting his Spanish at the City Colleges of Chicago, at night classes after his work day in their downtown classrooms. He also added practical use of street Spanish through various friends, particularly those on the volleyball courts. He would always laugh out loud when recalling the telltale chant that finished many of the matches, ¡Uno más! (clap-clap-clap), ¡Uno más! (clap-clap-clap), ¡Uno más! (clap-clap-clap), ¡Uno más! (clap-

clap-clap)...until of course the "one more" game-winning point was delivered...often by him on an "Ace serve" or with a strategic pass to a teammate near the net.

Ted's north-bound flight from Mexico was headed to Houston, the home of this year's National volleyball tournament of his international volleyball league. Ted's team was among the favorites in its division. Every year this prestigious tournament is staged in a different city, but this year's location fit quite well with his work obligations in León.

The teams came from all corners of North America. He reunited with many past opponents, many of whom he had known for several years and had made some lasting friendships. There would also be lots of new faces of future friends. I was more than just Ted's friend in that I served as the team's cheerleader and trainer. I was also his own live-in Spanish professor; I was a former full-time high school Spanish teacher in Indiana before going on to a career in travel training. We often communicated in Spanish on a daily basis to enhance both of our skills in the language.

As promised, I was right there at his gate as he made it through the jetway and into the terminal.

"How was the flight?"

Ben Dales and B. B. Beaudreaux

"It was great," Ted said. "The meal was pretty decent. I had the huachinango a la mexicana."

Red snapper, Mexican-style. "Good choice," I remarked.

"And I had a wonderful nap. We were flying in the clouds for most of it, but just before we landed I caught a glimpse of the Gulf coastline in Galveston. I saw the Johnson Space Center--"

"'Houston, we have a problem,'" I joked.

Ted laughed, grabbing me in a big hug.

"Do you think we have time this weekend to see it?" He asked. "You know how I've always said I would volunteer to be the first civilian in space."

I began excitedly talking about the rental car deal that I secured just a few minutes prior to his arrival. After landing early, I decided just for kicks to see how much it might cost to rent a car. Having learned that a taxi ride to the hotel would likely cost over $50 one way plus tip, I realized it would be best just to rent a car to get around Houston. We were looking forward to our three-day weekend together.

As we drove to our hotel, he continued describing his view to me of flying over the massive city of Houston. He told me he saw a domed stadium, a-ha! The Astrodome, although we both knew the hometown Astros no longer used it. He said he also saw the Astros' current home, an open-air stadium with a retractable roof option to offer protection from undesirable weather. We chuckled about whether that also referred to too much heat during August. We also wondered whether the Astros were in town, but then thought better of it. These tournaments are fun but certainly dominate one's time from morning into the night.

Before long, the weekend was well underway and the tournament began. His team placed a healthy 3rd after falling in overtime to the eventual champion in the division from Montreal. Everyone was happy with such a good showing, although of course it would have been nice to win it all. It soon became time to wish our friends a safe journey with promises to keep in touch until the start of next season's schedule at various cities around North America. Many left early to catch late flights home on Sunday night, undoubtedly to be able to arrive home (even if exhausted) to make a quick turn-around to work on Monday morning.

For us, however, there was no such late-night flight schedule. I had arranged a birthday addition for Ted to our fun weekend. On Monday morning we would be flying from Houston to Denver. Ted loved Colorado, especially downhill skiing. I made

Ben Dales and B. B. Beaudreaux

a reservation for three days at a dude ranch resort in Breckenridge. I knew this was a bit of a dream for him, to stay at a "cowboy place."

For Ted's birthday, I planned another dream of his--a whitewater rafting trip in the Breckenridge area. Ted watched this sport on TV and mentioned that he wanted to do it at least once during his life. Now it looked as if it would happen.

Even if I do say so myself, I was always very good at finding sentimental and meaningful little gifts and appropriate cards for so many occasions we had shared, but this promised gift of whitewater rafting would be by far the best. Before he shut his eyes to sleep on his birthday eve at the dude ranch, he told me he knew he was sure to dream about the great fun ahead starting in the morning of his birthday.

Before we knew it, it was morning. I had already been up to get a coffee and look outside, so I could share the "weather report" with him. It was indeed daylight, and I wished him a happy birthday in bed singing the traditional birthday song of México, Las Mañanitas. It was a perfect start, and also a bit of a birthday tradition between the two of us.

"Come here," I motioned him over to look out the window. "You just have to see what a beautiful day it is!"

At first glance, he did a double-take. Ted was speechless. Yes, it was the morning of his May 25 birthday, and most years, it was a wonderful spring-like day. What he observed today, though, was unbelievable. There had been an overnight blizzard. It was sunny outside, and there was over a foot of snow.

Whitewater rafting seemed to be out of the question. We wondered about downhill skiing?

CHAPTER 5

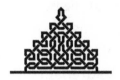

Ted: Surprise Powder Skiing

Absolutely breathtaking! Two feet of fresh powder from the night before, all light and airy. This was the type of snow that one expects to see in January when the temperatures are far below zero. Instead, it was May 25--my birthday--and I was on the highest-peak ski lift headed up to the west wall of the Arapahoe Basin. I could see the mountain town of Keystone below. Since the snowstorm during the night had cut off the power, the lifts were initially not able to run. All the locals, though, knew that Arapahoe had its own generator capable of powering up the lift I was now on. There were very few people on the slopes--it was, after all, a workday Tuesday.

The sun was bearing down and the warmth felt good on my face amidst the cool, post-blizzard Colorado air. Not having packed for (and thus a little unprepared for) such a surprise snowstorm, here I was attired in blue jeans, a medium-weight jacket, a baseball cap, and a pair of borrowed gloves from the ranch resort where we were staying. Since my falling down on the slopes was not expected to be an issue, there was no need to bundle up. The air was crisp and I caught a whiff of the rich aroma of pine needles and mountain air that just gets one's adrenaline flowing.

I got to the departure point of the ski lift and slid off early from the seat with my poles in one hand and skated my way over to the top of the rim. As I passed the ski lift operator, I happily gave a thumbs up. He was smiling from ear to ear. We knew having this kind of snow at this time of the year was a once-in-a-lifetime event.

I looked up to see the city of Breckenridge in the far-off distance, but no one else was on the mountain just then to share the view with me. Most of the staff had already left for the season. So just between me and the lift operators, plus perhaps only a dozen or so hardy and well-seasoned skiers, we had this beautiful powder-capped mountain all to ourselves. At that moment, my smile widened too.

As I poised to take the leap from the pinnacle of what is known as one of the most difficult double black diamond runs in Colorado, the west wall of Arapahoe Basin, my thoughts turned back to an

Ben Dales and B. B. Beaudreaux

earlier time back in my youth. I recalled how then I had been on top of this very peak well above the tree growth line with my high school best friend John, along with his brother Roger and their sister Erin. The three of us had skied this same mountain when we were all in our early twenties and had a blast together. I wished they were here with me now.

Back in the current moment again, I breezed down the mountain as I hugged every turn. I found myself leaning far back because of the huge amount of powder, flying over moguls and small cliffs, and zigzagging in and out of the glades areas (in skiing lingo, this means in and out of the trees). I kept thinking about how much fun I would have in relaying this story to all of my friends. An absolutely unexpected and unbelievable snowstorm swept in the night before, while I slept at a dude ranch in the mountains. I just happened to be in Colorado--on my birthday--which turned into one of the best ski adventure stories I could ever tell them. How in late May, I skied the same mountain I did almost ten years ago! I was able to conquer a full day of skiing one of the most challenging mountains in North America, and as it turned out, without a single fall.

On this momentous birthday, I found I was in better shape than ever before in my life.

CHAPTER 6

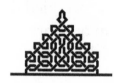

Ted: Making the Decision

Despite being an active, healthy athlete, I started experiencing a recurring pain in my lower back. Sometimes I would feel this pain all the way down into the left ankle. I noticed a small lump on my left calf. It seemed these pains were affecting my performance on the volleyball court.

The back pain came and went. When I increased my physical activity, I would often have more pain--an annoyance, but certainly not debilitating. If I took a week or two off from my physical routine, the pain would subside. However, it was difficult for me to take even a day or two off, since physical activity was a major part of my life. The pain in my ankle was constant. No matter what I did, this pain would not subside.

When I eventually mentioned it to my general physician, Dr. Lottens, he sent me to an orthopedic physician, Dr. Lars Clack.

Dr. Clack prescribed steroid shots but they did nothing to help the pain in my lower left leg and ankle.

He then ran me through a series of tests--both X-rays and MRIs. Cumbersome though it was, I submitted to whatever he suggested. A few months went by and I still had no answers. My patience started to wane with his next recommendation.

"Myelogram? Why do I need that?"

"So we can see inside your spinal column."

"Why exactly do you keep making me have these tests? You told me the steroid injections would stop the pain. The pain seems even worse now."

I thought back to the series of three steroid shots initially ordered for me to have as a hospital outpatient. Not only did I well remember those shots, I thought about the insurance dilemma created by having them. The bill I received by mail was incredulously expensive and my insurance company balked at paying for them. I encountered one of those "out of network" issues that so many of us have faced. In my case, I had previously made sure that the hospital was "in network." However, I later learned that the steroid injection physician was "out of network," something over which I had no control. It took several phone calls and endless documentation before I received partial payment coverage from the insurance company. These types of occurrences are classic "bait and switch" examples that patients are forced to experience.

"Ted, are you with me?"

I looked at Dr. Clack.

"You seemed to be in another world there. You were telling me about the pain being worse. I simply need to discover why you are in such pain."

"Well, I don't know why you didn't do the tests in the first place," I answered. "I mean--before you gave me the steroid injections, if you thought there might be more than one reason that my lower left leg and ankle are hurting?"

"Well, we thought at the time it was because of a pinched nerve."

"Yeah, but couldn't you confirm whether or not it was a pinched nerve before you did that series of injections on me? I must point out I seem worse than before I ever came to see you, Dr. Clack."

Ben Dales and B. B. Beaudreaux

"Yes, and I'm sorry, but if you have this myelogram, we will be able to link a direct cause of what is going on inside your spine. Your insurance will cover it, don't worry; we've already checked. I will have my nurse schedule you to have this done."

"Well, how exactly is it different from all the other tests you've done?"

"You see, in this test we inject dye directly into your dural sac--this is what houses your spinal cord. The fluid moves the dye around with the help of a machine that inverts you. The dye contrast is radioactive."

"WHAT?"

"It won't hurt you. It's only a low-level radioactive dye that disintegrates within a couple of hours."

"Well...then what?"

"Then, when you are inverted, we take a series of X-rays to see where the dye travels. It will tell us if there are any areas that need attention."

"Are you sure this will help you figure out what is going on? And what is this going to cost?" I didn't want to end up with another pile of bills.

"Don't worry, my office will make sure your insurance will cover everything except a small copay. We have the correct procedure codes already submitted to your insurance, and it's completely covered."

"Is it safe?"

"Ted, would I suggest anything that might hurt you?"

"I'm a lot worse off than when we started," I said.

"I know, but we will see what is happening inside."

I wanted to fix the problem, but this endless series of tests was getting me nowhere. I just wanted to get back to my daily life without the pain I was experiencing.

"Are there any risks?"

"The only one would be a little spinal fluid leakage, and that has rarely happened."

So I went back to the hospital.

They used huge needles to inject the dye inside my dura. While I hung upside-down during the X-rays, the pain escalated. Two hours afterwards, I had a horrible headache.

Ben Dales and B. B. Beaudreaux

I went back home to sink into my comfortable bed and the headache subsided somewhat. When I got up to get something to eat in the evening, the headache came back with ferocity.

The next day, I had to get up early for work. Three clients in different parts of the country were going to do upgrades on the same day. It would have been easier for me to do these installations in person, but the three clients believed they did not have the luxury of time, and neither did I.

After about an hour at my desk, the headache returned worse than the day before.

To try to alleviate the pain while guiding the upgrades, I literally laid on the floor with a different phone to each ear and three keyboards on the floor with me.

"What the heck is going on?" Our company owner, Harry, stopped in shock when he came by my office and saw me on the floor.

Covering both phone receivers, I whispered, "Harry, I can't talk. I'm upgrading our clients' computers and haven't quite finished."

"To hell with them," he said. "I'm calling an ambulance."

"No! No, wait, Harry. The last thing I want is to go to the hospital in an ambulance."

"You can't work on the floor, Ted. Something is definitely wrong. I'm scared of your being like this and trying to work."

"But the clients..."

"Forget about the clients! They'll just have to wait. Now, let me call the ambulance."

"No. No. Have Dick drive me home, or better yet, have him follow me in his car, and then I'll get my neighbor, Cora...you remember her? She's a doctor, she can drive me to the hospital."

"Are you sure?"

"Yes, but please don't call the ambulance."

"Teddy, we need you, but first we need you to be well. We've gotten you the best damn insurance in the world. Use it."

"Okay, Harry. I'll go to the hospital," I promised.

At the hospital, I was ushered from the emergency room (ER) into the operating room (OR). As it turned out, the myelogram left a hole in my dura, one through which it was leaking spinal fluid. This led to a diminished amount of pressure in my brain stem, causing the terrible spinal headache. Blood was drawn from my arm with a rather large syringe, and then it was injected as needed to the site of the myelogram puncture. This was to act as a patch. The blood was supposed to clot around the hole and stop the leaking of spinal fluid.

During the injection part, I passed out.

When I awoke, the OR doctor was telling me that this should work, but that this was only the theory of how the patch was to work. She further advised that if I still had the spinal headache later, I was to return to the hospital to be admitted.

She then paused before emphasizing, "No activity whatsoever. You are to go home, and not do anything."

"That's easier said than done when you live by yourself, Doctor."

"Don't you have family?"

"None that are helpful in my house. My good friend Deni is out of town."

"What about your doctor friend who brought you here?"

"Yes, she would be willing to help me, but I just hate having to keep asking her for favors all the time."

"Well, if you don't have anyone at home, you will have to stay in the hospital."

"Okay, okay." I definitely did not want that. "Could you have someone bring her in her from the waiting room?"

My friend and neighbor, Dr. Cora Lane, of course agreed to help me. She did a good job, but she also had her practice to run and her own life to live, too. There was no romance between us, but we cared about each other all the same. I was glad to have a good neighbor.

I was also glad I had a good boss. Harry insisted that I not return to work for the rest of the week. Nevertheless, I was getting calls from clients at home (some of them I had given my home number for "emergencies") and it was difficult for me to stay away from my work. While I was recuperating, I dialed in on a few systems to fix some issues that had crept up for clients.

The Diagnosis

Dr. Clack put me through an entire series of tests. The analyzed results determined that I had a condition known as Spondylolisthesis, a so-called congenital condition. It was explained as a situation wherein the last vertebrae before the sacrum was slightly forward in its positioning from what was considered "normal" for a straight spinal column. Although estimates reveal that a high percentage of the human population has some degree of this type of anomaly, its effect on people varies greatly. Some have no problem with this condition, while others have severe back trouble associated with it, all dependent on a variety of factors. Among these factors could be how active a person is...or how inactive. It also depends upon the degree of how offset the placement of the vertebrae actually is.

"Spondylolisthesis is the cause of your recurring back problem and the pain in your left ankle," Dr. Clack confirmed. "I recommend a spinal fusion. This is the cure you need to stop the pain, and it should also prevent any similar pains in the future."

When Dr. Clack came to me with the suggestion of a spinal fusion, he stated this to me with complete confidence that the fusion would entirely eradicate the issue causing the nerve leading to my left leg to become irritated. Additionally, I did my own research as to others who had this type of surgery. I read about many who did find that it permanently relieved them of their back pain. Some had found relief in their sciatica too.

As for me, I was young, active, and lived a very health-conscious lifestyle. Dr. Clack even told me that because I was healthy and active, the fusion of the L5 (lumbar, the last free vertebrae in the spinal column) to the S1 (sacrum) was guaranteed to work.

He also told me that he was going to make it virtually impossible for me not to fuse by using the latest technology that was proven to make bone matter grow fast. This technology, unbeknownst to me at the time, was my first introduction to this particular medical device manufacturing company, TREND Electronic Medical Device Manufacturers.

TREND was promoting a device for fusions called a "bone growth stimulator," specifically for fusions like the one Dr. Clack proposed. The bone growth stimulator resembled two large watch batteries that had four wire leads with terminal endings designed to be placed near where the fusion was to take place, at the point of the spinous processes between the L5 and S1. Dr. Clack insisted at the time that not only would my body fuse the area naturally just as it would a broken bone, but that this device would "electrically stimulate" the area, which in turn was to enhance the growth of bone.

The fusion itself he described as routine. He professed that the chances of this surgery not helping were next to none. The implant of this

Ben Dales and B. B. Beaudreaux

device, he said, would guarantee that the fusion would take place. He also stated that because I had "good" insurance, it meant that payment coverage could include this device that would ensure the fusion.

I was full of questions about my upcoming surgery and thus wrote them all down on a long list, so that I could ask him everything that might otherwise be forgotten during our office visits. I would always update my own personal medical journal, in which I recorded as much as I could at every appointment, with every doctor. This is why I have such a complete record of what happened during this time in my life.

Among the questions I asked him was "Have you ever had an unsuccessful fusion?"

"No, never," said Dr. Clack.

"How painful is it to have fusions?"

As he offered answers to my line of questioning, he started telling me of other patients who had undergone the surgery.

"Well, some people are up and walking right after surgery," he responded. "Some spend the night in the hospital, but usually they go home within a couple of days. A removable body cast must be worn to keep everything in line for six weeks while the fusion takes hold, but you should be back on the volleyball court within six months."

"In fact," he continued, "the most painful part patients complain about is the extraction of the donor bone that comes from the hip. But with your insurance and the bone growth stimulator, we might not have to extract bone from your hip. Instead, we can use the bone that filters out during the laminectomy, which is the routing out of the transforaminal canal where the nerve comes out of the spinal column. There is a blood/bone filter that will allow me to use this bone instead of extracting it from your posterior pelvic girdle. That and the bone growth stimulator will ensure that you have a solid strong fusion from the L5 to the sacrum."

"And because you are in such fine shape, I think you will bounce back from this in no time at all."

Ben Dales and B. B. Beaudreaux

CHAPTER 7

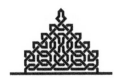

Deni: Making the Decision

When Ted started complaining about the pain extending from his back and especially down into his left leg, I was empathetic. I noticed the pain would happen following periods of physical activity, especially during and after his frequent volleyball competitions. I was not then nor am I now a masseuse, but I administered back and leg massages whenever this happened and they seemed to help, if only for a short time. However, after a while, the massages were no longer providing enough relief.

"You need to tell the doctor about the pain," I said.

Ted was resistant at first, but when the pain refused to subside, he went to see our primary doctor. We realized he would likely be referred to a specialist, as had been my experience in the past with our doctor. The referrals had been reliable ones, including my orthopedic surgeon who had completed surgery for permanent repair of my dislocated shoulder using a titanium prong.

The referral led us to a specialist, Dr. Lars Clack, working out of the same partnership of doctors as my orthopedic surgeon. Although we had no other knowledge about this new specialist doctor, we at least could vouch for the fact that my surgery from that office and from a partner doctor to him had gone well and completely stopped my shoulder from dislocating.

Ted went alone to see this doctor during the daytime while I was at work. He returned with the advice that he might have to consider a spinal surgery to remedy and repair his pain problems. He was encouraged to think about it, and to pursue getting a second opinion if he wanted. The doctor did instill a level of confidence and Ted even mentioned that this doctor carried a rather fatherly demeanor about him at this first appointment.

Ted thought about it and ended up making another appointment with this specialist surgeon to discuss the idea of spinal surgery in more depth. Ted again went alone to this second appointment.

"Well, the doctor assured me it would be a routine surgery," he said. "He even said I'd be right

Ben Dales and B. B. Beaudreaux

back on the volleyball court within six months."

Ted did in fact go for a second opinion prior to going under the knife. The neurologist he chose to see for a second opinion, Dr. Lanzler, was also from a referral, but the meeting with this second-opinion doctor did not go well. Ted came back home to state that this doctor was gruff at best and did not seem to have very much time to devote to Ted's situation. This neurologist only listened to Ted's story and then proceeded to take all of thirty seconds to tell him not to do any surgery.

Dr. Lanzler instead recommended more physical therapy. Ted countered that as an athlete, he already had been doing all kinds of physical therapy. He was always very active in non-contact sports, because he had seen repeatedly what could happen in the more violent sports like football, soccer, and even baseball. He had made competitive volleyball his primary sports option.

Therefore, we opted for Ted to go with the advice of the first doctor and proceed with the surgery. Prior to this decision, we had also considered the option of whether to proceed with the surgery at that very time or whether to delay it for an international trip we might take. In my job I had received a travel benefit that would allow us to travel to Asia. We specifically were trying to plan a trip to China and Thailand. As attractive as this trip sounded to us, I was the one who was leery about it. I knew how much and how often Ted's pain was recurring. I could only envision something going awry during the trip and seeing it result in his being confined in some Chinese hospital. I too trusted and believed the doctor recommending the surgery. I took to heart what we were being told about the projected recovery time. It seemed sensible to take the trip after Ted's recovery, so that he could truly enjoy himself on such an exotic trip destination. After all, Ted was all but guaranteed to recuperate completely within a few months.

In a nutshell, this is what led Ted, and me with him, into that hospital for the surgery--ironically on the Presidential Election Day of 2000, November 7.

We had no idea that day would change our lives forever, as well as that of our country and the world.

Ben Dales and B. B. Beaudreaux

CHAPTER 8

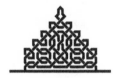

Ted: The Day of Surgery and the Aftermath

What the hell happened?

Dr. Clack told me the spinal-fusion surgery was going to be almost like an outpatient procedure, and he made the recovery seem like it would be a "walk in the park." He told me I would be able to go back home as early as the very next day.

I could barely move.

I hit the morphine button so many times. The pain was searing. The nurses adjusted the dosage three times.

Still no relief.

A few days later, I developed a very severe infection. During the second night, I started sweating profusely. The infection was virulent and out of control.

My general practitioner, Dr. Lottens, started coming to the hospital every day to see me and monitor the infection. By the fourth day, not only was Dr. Lottens visiting me, but so too was his newest partner, Dr. England. Dr. Clack was seeing me every day too. The look in his eyes made me wonder if this recovery was not going as planned.

Dr. England took a clinical, no-nonsense approach when he was questioning me about what he thought might be causing this virulent infection. He asked me about my sexual proclivities and was extremely blatant about whether I had ever had sex with "anyone" without using a condom. Of course having grown up during the time period I had, I was fully aware of the HIV epidemic and had never, ever taken a chance with even my most trusted lovers.

I had seen so many friends' lives upended after becoming parents too early that I was not about to jeopardize my career and become a father before I was ready. Although I did plan on having a family, I knew that option would have to be delayed until later in my life so that I could fully engage my career and have enough money to send my children to college. I had also been influenced by observing the myriad of poor people in the areas

Ben Dales and B. B. Beaudreaux

where I traveled while working as a consultant in Latin America. I knew that if I had the chance to start a family, the children would be adopted. There were simply too many people in the world living on the edge, and I knew that there would always be neglected children who need a good home.

Dr. England insisted that I have an HIV test. It took a few days to get the results, but I knew that my results would be negative. Yet, the severity of the infection really made me wonder if somehow I contracted some other type of disease. The results came back negative, and once again, the doctors were perplexed as my infection would not subside.

The fever persisted despite the strong antibiotics pumped into me daily. The nurses were changing my bedding three or four times a night as it repeatedly became soaked with sweat. As the days went on, I had no appetite.

Six nights later, my fever finally broke, and I was able to eat some food. I had a catheter in me for that whole time, another detail of which the doctor forgot to inform me before going into this surgery. I was actually glad that I did, because I could hardly move without being in horrible pain, let alone get up and out of bed to use the bathroom.

But after the fever finally broke, the nurses--and God bless them--encouraged me to try to get out of bed. I asked them to take the catheter out; actually this was more like making a deal, because I told them if it was out, then I would be forced to get up to urinate. They concurred with the deal and with the help of two nurses, I learned to use the walker to get up and walk to the bathroom.

At this point, after many conversations with the nurses, I had come to the conclusion that just being in the hospital was subjecting me to more and more virulent bacteria that could cause infection. I asked if I could be released to go home. I was told that I could but only if I had a nurse at home, which I was gladly willing to pay for. To get me home, I needed an ambulance, because riding upright in a car was out of the question. Therefore, this was another condition of my being released. However, it was finally agreed that since my sister had a full-sized pleasure van, she along with two of my friends would get me into the van and back to my home.

CHAPTER 9

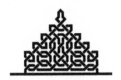

Deni: The Day of Surgery and the Day After

It was November 7, 2000, the date of the presidential election. It was also--more importantly to us--the date of Ted's spinal fusion surgery. It was a partial work day for me in downtown Chicago. I wanted to take off the entire day to be at the hospital, but as it turned out, the corporate concerns of my company overruled that possibility. I was scheduled to fly out to corporate headquarters in suburban Denver later that evening, so I would be required to check in at the office during the afternoon to review last-minute details of our upcoming two days of meetings.

I got up early to go vote right after the polls opened at 6 a.m., while Ted was at home getting ready. He had voted absentee ahead of time. I proceeded to take Ted to the hospital on Chicago's

North Side located over twenty miles away from our home. I stayed there throughout the bulk of the morning until Ted was wheeled away into surgery. At this point, I made my leave and took Chicago's "El" train downtown to the office located in the heart of the Loop.

Even though I had been advised the surgery would take over four hours and that he would not be coherent until later in the afternoon, I still called the hospital several times just to be sure. Somewhere around 3 p.m., I was able to "escape" the office with all that would be needed for Denver. I would not be going home prior to my late evening flight from O'Hare.

Upon arrival at the hospital, I was informed Ted was still not out of surgery. The predicted four-hour surgery was taking longer--as it turned out, it took six hours. By the time I got to see him it was already getting dark out (clocks had already "fallen back").

Ted's appearance brought tears to my eyes. It was evident he was in much pain. He looked as if he'd been through the literal wringer.

Even so, he inquired about the election. We turned on the television in his room to check into what was going on with the vote counts. Announcers on all major networks were predicting a late night, as the race was neck-and-neck. Our home state of Illinois had long since been declared for Democrat Al Gore, the incumbent Vice President, but many of the bordering states appeared either too close to call or had already been chalked up for Republican challenger George W. Bush.

We continued to watch and make small talk, in between Ted's short little naps caused by the pain medication he had been given. He was still connected to an IV, so hospital dining in his room was not an option. Finally, at around 8 p.m., I unfortunately had to say my goodbyes and drive to O'Hare for my late flight out.

How I wished I could be with Ted, not only for the obvious reason of lending moral and whatever other support I could to his recovery, but also due to the fact that we had always discussed politics. I wondered how he was doing and what he was thinking about all that was going on.

I proceeded to shower and dress for the day's meetings, to be held at corporate headquarters outside Denver. However, I was simultaneously experiencing a seemingly small but irritating problem. I apparently had something lodged in my right eye and could not get it out. I washed both eyes, but to no avail. It was a painful nuisance and inhibited my eyesight from that eye. Even so, I decided to attempt to deal with it and took the hotel shuttle to the meetings.

During the first round of meetings, it continued to worsen. I had no idea what was going on; this was new territory to me. By midday, I decided to return home to my own long-time doctor. Whatever was going on was more than frightening to me by now. I suffered through the long shuttle ride back to the new Denver International Airport, located rather far away from downtown, unlike the old, convenient Stapleton Airport. During the flight, it was not any better – in fact, it got worse. Not getting back into O'Hare until late afternoon on that Wednesday, I drove with one good eye directly to my doctor's office, where I had already phoned ahead. He took one quick look and referred me to an ophthalmologist downtown. This doctor listened to my story, taking in where I had been, and immediately determined I had been a victim of Denver dry air. The dry air in the famous Mile-High City had literally caused my eyelid to scratch the cornea of my eye. He gave me some soothing and moisturizing solutions, which helped a bit, and sent me off with a couple of samples and some prescriptions to fill later.

Already feeling relief, I headed immediately to the hospital to see Ted. Still a bit out of it due to

Ben Dales and B. B. Beaudreaux

pain medication, he took one look at me and asked whether it had already been two days. I smiled and said no, that I had come back early to see him and take care of him. I did not tell him about my dry air eye problem until later.

We began talking and talking about how he was doing, about what the surgeon had said (and not said), and about the goofy election goings-on. Already it was being predicted that the election results might not be determined even by the January 20 inauguration. Little did we know that he might be on the road to recovery before the country would be.

CHAPTER 10

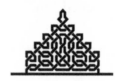

Ted: Home Again for Recuperation

I really had a good support system. Deni was going to stay with me and be able to commute to work on the METRA train. Deni, who was Lead Trainer for one of Chicago's largest corporate travel management firms had saved enough PTO (Paid Time Off) to be able to stay home during my first week of recuperation.

I felt so lucky that Deni was going to be able to take care of me. While lying in bed all those hours, I tried to think up a list of my other friends or family members who would have been so--well, not just insistent on helping someone like me in my present condition, but assisting someone who could barely manage getting out of bed. Yes, Deni was wanting to stay with me in order that I might recover quickly. I soon realized that the list I tried to think of in my head was short. In fact, there was only one person on that list--Deni!

In spite of its prestigious location, my home was not grandiose at all. It was a rather small Craftsman bungalow that I had painstakingly restored to its original modest but elegant state. My bedroom, the largest of two, was relatively small. To the credit of William Radford, the architect who designed this home built in 1911, it had two sets of double pane windows--one facing south and one facing west. However, for my projected recovery time, I had arranged for a hospital bed (on loan from my next door neighbor Cora) to be set up in the large family room with lots of windows facing north and east. It also had its own private bathroom adjacent to it.

On the day I was brought home, I dwelled on the fact that I would be recuperating in this large room and that is when it hit me. I really wanted to be in my own room, even if smaller, due to its plethora of sunlight coming through the south windows and then later in the day from the west. Adding to this was a magnificent garden just outside the windows. The lot itself was huge by city standards (50' by 180'). When I purchased the home and moved in just four years before, there was very little growing in the lot save for the trees, a few shrubs, and some rather sickly grass.

I, along with Deni's help, had worked hard to turn the lot into a gardening showcase, good enough to be invited to be on the annual Beverly Hills Garden Walk for several years. I was especially proud of the garden design I had drawn up and implemented. Although it was already autumn, the yard was beautiful to look at with all the varied species, conifers, and countless other plants that were flowing and ornamental. I knew that, if anything, being able to enjoy the garden view from my recuperation room would only help me get better.

As I stayed in my preferred bedroom, it was Deni who was sleeping in the back room hospital bed. My home's second bedroom was already being occupied by my father, for whom I had become caregiver after I bought the house.

Deni became the primary caregiver for both of us, at least until I could recuperate enough to reassume that role for my father. It was at this point that I realized Deni was so much more than a good friend--Deni was truly my soulmate. Although I felt a bit selfish to myself about all the time and effort Deni was putting in to my recovery, I couldn't help but think how much of a struggle it would have been not to have anyone in my life at that time. As it turned out, Deni simply never really moved out as our relationship continued

Ben Dales and B. B. Beaudreaux

to develop. The Craftsman bungalow became the home we shared together.

After that surgery, I did exactly as I was told by the surgeon who performed it. I wore a body cast which kept everything in alignment. Because I was practically immobile, I did not do much of anything except visit the doctor. The entire ordeal was perplexing and left me truly dumbfounded, as the doctor's optimism led me to believe that I would be up and walking around so quickly after surgery.

Cora came over every day to make sure everything was going well. Even so, the recovery seemed to take forever. The days rolled by slowly, and I was on a lot of pain medication. I was sleeping up to eighteen hours a day and seemed only to be alert when going to the bathroom. I was also trying to transition from a soft diet back to regular food. Since I was in bed this whole time, I never could have done it without the help of people who made sure I was eating, drinking, and bathing. It helped immensely for me to be able to get around during my recuperation, once I was able to manage picking myself up using my arm strength and the walker that had been provided for me. Still, the going was rough, to say the least.

The one constant comfort I had during the entire first month was that every time I woke up, my very tiny and extremely fluffy cat, Blueberry, was lying on the edge of the bed next to me. She knew that something was wrong, and somehow having that wonderful gaze staring at me every time I opened my eyes gave me much-needed comfort.

By the time I was due for my next doctor's appointment, I was able to sit upright but still had to be driven to the hospital. Dr. Clack was optimistic. More X-rays were taken, and he seemed to think that everything was "in place." He showed me the X-rays and pointed out where the battery pack and lead wires were placed, explaining why they were in the position they were. The "lump" of the battery did not bother me so much, and this gave me hope that even if I didn't fuse naturally, the battery pack would ensure complete fusion.

Harry, my boss, called me many times during the first two months I was off work.

"Just concentrate on healing," he'd reassure me. "Your position will always be secure here."

All the clients asking for me were told that I was temporarily on short-term disability. As the cards, flowers, gifts, and calls poured in, Harry made sure the company was forwarding them to my home (assuredly in hopes of speeding along my recuperation). After three months off, I was

Ben Dales and B. B. Beaudreaux

still on the payroll and receiving my full pay and benefits and even my bonuses.

There were a few clients from Latin America calling me at home to ask me if I wanted to come to various places where the weather was warm and where I could recuperate faster. Some of them were even telling me that they wanted me to come to work for them, since my skills had saved them from ruin when I was able to complete all the necessary upgrades prior to the Y2K debacle. Little did they know I was having an unknown debacle going on in my back at the time. I was very gracious to all of them, but I told everyone (speaking in Spanish) I had to follow doctor's orders and start physical therapy to get me back to work as soon as possible. There was never any feeling by me that my career was anything but stable. I knew I would be welcomed back anytime.

The visits and the X-rays continued, and the fusion was taking place on the right side of the spinal processes, but not on the left. After six weeks, the bone was still not filling in where it should have been on the left side of the area that needed to be fused. Over time, whenever I stood upright, I was in even greater pain that I was before the surgery.

I had been on pain medication ever since returning home from the hospital, but my dosages were low. I was taking just two Vicodin a day and sometimes, especially when I was in a prone position or lying down (my only way to be comfortable), I would only need to take one. In spite of this, I found that I needed to take two every time I had to stand up for any length of time, because that is when the pain in my left leg was prohibitive.

I continued to stay in bed most of the time until the incision healed. I started going to physical therapy as a recommended part of my recuperation. I began slowly at first. After about three months, I started to get nervous. There was no improvement in my condition.

The doctor ordered X-rays every time I returned to his office without really explaining the results.

"Keep doing physical therapy," Dr. Clack told me after every visit.

"I am, Doc. I'm doing everything the physical therapists are telling me to do, but every time I am in an upright position, my leg is in horrible pain," I would explain. "I'm limited in what I can do during therapy. It's always on a mat on the floor."

After one such visit, he asked me if I would consider hydrotherapy. I agreed wholeheartedly, having been a swimmer and diver all my life. I

Ben Dales and B. B. Beaudreaux

would be back on familiar turf, to say the least.

Everyone like me who lives in Chicago and pays property taxes knows that the Chicago Park District (aka "Parks and Recreation" everywhere else) are a substantial part of one's personal property tax assessment. The payoff for citizens is the numerous public swimming pools located throughout the city. My closest pool was in a park district less than a five-minute drive from my home, and I had friends bring me there every day.

Being in the water took the pressure off my spine and thus off the nerve that led to my left leg. The pain seemed to be less intense when my body was floating, so I began going to my neighborhood pool every day of the week for the next year and a half. While doing laps in the pool with my goggles and bathing cap on, I would stare at the bottom where the lap line is painted and think to myself, Ted, every lap you make gets you a step closer to getting back to your career and onto the volleyball court.

CHAPTER 11

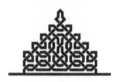

Deni: Home Again for Recuperation

This was new territory in our relationship. Never before had we been on less than equal footing when it came to physical capabilities. Granted, each of us had occasionally fallen temporarily ill with colds or sore throats or even flu. I had undergone a couple of surgeries myself, but still had not been in long-term need of recuperative care. This was going to be the first type of major recuperation we were going to experience between us.

In preparation for Ted's return from the hospital, I had stocked up the pantry with more food than usual in order that my trips out of the house would be kept to a minimum. I planned to use vacation time from work, so being home with him during the day would not be an issue. Finally, I stocked up on reading materials for him at home, hopefully to help his recuperative time pass better and more quickly.

After the nearly six days in the hospital following Ted's spinal surgery, the return home was a welcome one for both of us. For him, it was the obvious--getting away from sick people and bland food. During his time in the hospital environment, he had even managed to catch an infection. Going home meant leaving these kinds of possibilities behind him.

For me it meant not only having him back home where he belonged, but also it eliminated my going to the North Side hospital some twenty miles away through heavy Chicago traffic both ways. It eliminated my spending day after day at the hospital, my coming to his home each night to rifle through his closet and dresser drawers to find clean lounging clothes for him to wear--or failing that, washing and drying the dirty ones brought home. This was necessary especially during his period of infection, as he had developed such severe sweating that the nurses were forced to change his bed clothes almost hour after hour during the overnights. Of course I would not have had it any other way than going daily to the hospital, as I truly wanted to be with him during those first days of recuperation to do whatever I could to advocate for him with the staff and to lift his spirits as much as possible.

We asked his sister to drive us home from the hospital in her van that had seats that could completely recline, in order that the ride back home would not enhance his pain. His mom was also able to accompany us on this trip, a good thing given that she had been unable to make it to the hospital to see him there. The use of the van was especially important in that we could not preplan the time of day when his release would happen. We wanted to be doubly prepared in the event it would happen during the twice-daily traffic nightmare known as Chicago's rush hours. This was a good move as traffic was somewhat heavy and slow during our return to his Beverly Hills Chicago neighborhood. Upon our arrival home, we slowly and carefully helped him out of the van and onto the sidewalk to proceed at a slight elevation up and into the house.

My next pressing goal was to offer him a delectable meal to help compensate for all those subpar hospital meals he had endured (as had I, even if in the hospital cafeteria each day...there were no nearby quality eateries within walking distance of this particular hospital).

Now, this is a small but important detail: I had not been, nor was I ever going to be, anything close to a culinary whiz in the kitchen. Actually,

Ben Dales and B. B. Beaudreaux

my specialty is more like serving snack crackers garnished with Cheese Whiz and a slice of sweet black or Spanish green olives. (Although I do slice those olives myself!) Truth be known, he was the primary "chef" of the two of us, while I was the "bottle washer." We still share a humorous story with our friends about the time early in our relationship that he prepared a scrumptious meal for me (one of many to come throughout the coming years), and I complimented him by telling him, "You are a great cook." He immediately corrected me in a slightly haughty manner by saying, "I am not a cook. I am a chef." I never made that mistake again!

So there I was, in the position of becoming both the cook and bottle washer. Fortunately, one habit I followed throughout the years was putting together a collection of cookbooks of many genres. From these I had preplanned many options for all three daily meals. As it turned out, he was immensely grateful for my efforts and usually ate what I prepared with relish. Of course, he had grown vastly tired of boring hospital food options.

Thus we began the slow journey of Ted's recuperation. We had the first follow-up appointment the following week with his surgeon, but in the meantime we were on our own. There was one other major home factor to help him along in the meantime. This was the "love of his life" cat he had named Blueberry. In so many ways, the two of them were already the most loyal and loving of friends. Therefore, once Ted returned home and planted himself in his own bed, Blueberry immediately joined him to let him know how much he had been missed. The difference this time, though, was that Blueberry rarely left his side during the recuperative weeks to follow, except for the necessary trips to her litter box. Even getting her to leave in order to eat was a challenge on some days. Blueberry instinctively knew her daddy was in pain and needed her in the worst way. The measure of such help during recuperation can of course never be known, but it was easy to determine that this cat's devoted presence was certainly valuable.

The first appointment with the surgeon one week after his hospital departure came and went. Ted's progress had been minimal, as far as we were able to determine, and his surgical doctor had little to add other than a plea for patience. The many subsequent appointments with this same doctor were not much different or better.

Suffice it to say that Ted had gradually and readily ascertained that all was not well. He had been unable to recover to play competitive volleyball in "just six months" as his doctor had promised. He was unable even to return to work. Ted tried to work from home, but it was impossible for him to complete any work due to the discomfort and pain of sitting stationary for any longer than twenty minutes at a time.

His doctor's remedy at the time was prescription pain medication, as his pain was increasingly unbearable. Over time many different medications were employed, but the pain was not going away. Even after his surgery wound healed, the amount of pain he had to endure in his left leg did not diminish in the least. In fact, it was much worse.

Other than medication, the other recourse offered by his surgeon was physical therapy. However, instead of having a full-fledged consultation about Ted's situation and condition following his failed surgery, the doctor simply issued a referral. As a result, the physical therapist assigned to him demanded that he do activities that served as a detriment more than anything. A prime example was putting Ted on a stationary bicycle. Not only was this activity extremely painful to his already painful condition, it contributed to more physical harm to him. The therapist quickly became irked with Ted's inability to do this, seeming to read it instead as mere stubbornness on Ted's part. Eventually this mode of physical therapy came to an end, but it only happened after all those concerned came to realize why.

The real truth is that his long-term ability to walk came into question. He turned back to swimming, and it was the pool that prevented his inevitable inability to walk. He began an almost daily swimming routine at the local Chicago Park District pool within walking distance to his home. Although the original physical therapy as prescribed by his surgeon and other physicians proved to be ineffective, this therapeutic physical activity done over a near two-year time span proved to be the saving grace that maintained his ability to be upright and mobile. His determination had won out this time. Nevertheless, the pain in his left leg was a hundred times worse now than before the surgery.

What was Ted's prognosis--no one could tell us. The truth would reveal itself along the way.

CHAPTER 12

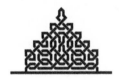

Ted: All Messed Up

After about six months, I called my surgeon's office and left a message with the nurse. "Hi this is Ted, I'm calling about the bone growth battery pack that is still subcutaneously implanted in my back. I want to find out how long it is supposed to stay there. Please give me a call back."

The physician assistant (P.A.) called me back. "That unit needs to remain in place for at least six to eight weeks, as that is how long it takes for the fusion to harden up."

"Did you say six to eight weeks?" I was incredulous.

"Yes, that's correct."

What I told her next totally silenced her.

"Well, I had my surgery around seven months ago. What is going on?"

After checking my records for accuracy, she told me she would inform Dr. Clack right away and that he would be in touch with me soon. I was finally going to be able to confront Dr. Clack about what was actually going on.

There was a message from Dr. Clack waiting on the answering machine when I arrived home from the pool.

"I am so sorry, Ted. We should have scheduled you to have the battery pack removed months ago. I'll schedule the appointment and set everything up. Please call."

After the battery was surgically removed from my back approximately five months after it was supposed to be removed, I found myself in Dr. Clack's office for a follow-up appointment. I asked him to show me the X-rays before and after the removal. I wanted to compare the X-rays of my spine with the battery-powered bone growth unit still in my back with how the ones taken after its removal looked.

"As you can see, Ted, the bone fusion has taken place here," he said, gesturing to the right side of my spine in the X-rays.

I could see, however, that the same growth had not taken place on the left side.

"What about the left side, why isn't the same growth happening there?"

"It could be the angle of the X-ray. We just have to give it more time," Dr. Clack assured me.

What was not told to me during my many trips back to my surgeon doctor's office was that the left side of the fusion was never going to fuse if it had not grown bone in that area by then. I had no way of knowing what was going on in my doctor's head, since he shared nothing about this. He simply left the bone growth stimulator in my back, apparently hoping it would eventually work.

I started getting more anxious at the lack of progress with the pain and healing, and Dr. Clack knew it. At this point, it had been months and months of X-rays, logjams, MRIs, and CTs; tests after tests but still no answers.

I told Dr. Clack my concerns about possibly losing my position at work, and he wrote a letter to my boss stating I was not yet being released to return to work. He changed my medication from Vicodin to Norco (at double the strength of the Vicodin I was taking). He additionally wanted me to see a neurologist at a major hospital in Chicago for a few tests. Dr. Clack told me that he would reassess everything in a few more months.

"What about swimming therapy?"

"Yes, keep swimming. That's the best physical therapy you possibly could be doing."

While back in the pool and staring at the same "lap line" back and forth every day, I once again kept to my mantra of saying to myself: "Ted, every lap gets you one step closer to returning to the volleyball court and back to your job, which you have missed so much."

Unbelievably, my boss Harry, having received the letter from Dr. Clack, kept me on a disability status with my health insurance intact. He even still sent me my annual bonus and assured me, as his wife Libby did, that I would always have a job within their corporation.

My teammates from my volleyball team continued calling me all the time and asking when I'd return, telling me their new setter had nowhere near the finesse I did. They told me they were no longer winning any of the tournaments they were participating in without me and encouraged me at least to come to watch. Hard to admit, I knew that even watching them on the court would be too emotional for me, seeing them all having fun

Ben Dales and B. B. Beaudreaux

together. I also quietly realized that without me on the court with them, our team was actually losing its backbone--the setter is the one who calls all the plays it runs on offense. I guess I was a bit fearful they would look at me on the sidelines as someone who had let them down. It was so ironic to me that as the former "backbone" of that team, I truly was the one being left behind. Although I didn't know it at the time, I was never going to return to be the backbone of my team and never again return to the court because of what I can now say was literally my own "broken backbone."

CHAPTER 13

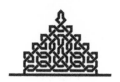

Deni: Looking for Answers

We had high hopes, yet a steadily increasing amount of impatience. Our high hopes were based on what his surgeon Dr. Clack had practically guaranteed--success. The near promise that Ted would be back at work--and back on the competitive volleyball circuit--within six months was constantly on our minds. However, also on our minds was the obvious: he was not getting one bit better. In fact, the pain and other related problems were on the rise.

During each of the subsequent follow-up appointments with Dr. Clack, we brought up our fears that all was not well and Ted was not on a proper recuperative path.

"All of this will take time," Dr. Clack explained. "The recovery will happen in its own due course."

Every time we returned to this doctor's office, we came away a little less optimistic. The healing was going much more slowly than we expected. Each time, the doctor begged for our patience with it and kept advising us to continue following the recommended recuperation protocol.

The doctor himself eventually expressed concern that the fusing was not happening as expected, at least not in any complete manner--he assured us it was proceeding fine on one side but not the other. Even so, I recall his plea that we continue our patience and the protocol. Finally, there came the fateful day when he seemed to admit he could do no more, but failed to give us any practical advice in what our next step should be.

Dr. Clack stated he had no more explanation of why Ted was experiencing even more pain than before his surgery. Dr. Clack admitted after more than a year that he could offer Ted no more help.

After all this frustrating time, we gradually came to realize that the surgery had not worked.

We were left lost and wandering. We meandered back into the office of our trusted primary physician, Dr. Lottens, who had referred us to this very surgeon doctor in the first place. Although extremely empathetic, our doctor and friend could offer no concrete answers or even suggestions. He began by advising us to continue to listen to Dr. Clack and to follow what he was telling us to do. After a few such appointments (and after recognizing our increasing levels of perplexed frustration), he did agree with us that perhaps it would not hurt to consult with another surgeon from another practice.

He gave us two referrals for consultation. The first one brought us back to Dr. Lanzler. If you recall, this was the "second opinion doctor" Ted had seen prior to his surgery with Dr. Clack. Yes, that's right--the one with the terrible bedside manner and no time to talk.

The return to Dr. Lanzler's office proved that not much had changed. The first words out of this physician's mouth were delivered in a forceful yell.

"You did it anyway, huh?"

The brief conversation that followed only produced some physical therapy sheets for Ted to take home and a pronouncement that he was unable to help any further. One thing noticeably missing from Dr. Lanzler's consultation was any admission that using the bone growth stimulator device during the first surgery had been a mistake.

Ben Dales and B. B. Beaudreaux

The other referral was for Dr. Shep Allen, a noted neurologist. Our consultation with him was a more congenial meeting than with Dr. Lanzler, even if no more productive. Dr. Allen's demeanor included a measure of empathetic listening that was refreshing and needed at this point. However, also missing from this initial consultation with Dr. Allen was any conversation that reflected that Dr. Clack erred by relying and putting so much trust in this relatively "new" device that was being promoted by TREND Electronic Medical Device Manufacturers in using the bone growth stimulator device.

Nevertheless, Ted did come away with the name of another physician to see. This was Dr. Doug Feisler.

Consultations with Dr. Feisler were not any easier than those with Lanzler or Allen, as they forced Ted to again relive all that had transpired and the pain involved. Dr. Feisler did understand eventually, though, that something could and must be done to rectify the condition in which Ted was living.

He recommended a second surgery, one vastly different from the first in that it was guaranteed to be more difficult and likely more painful.

This surgery was to involve literally undoing the first surgery and starting all over. It meant Dr. Feisler would need to start with the side of the fusion that did actually work. He would be removing all that fused bone on the right side of the spinal column in order to ensure that both sides of the fusion would be intact. This was also the only way, he stated, that the bones could be aligned correctly in Ted's spine.

CHAPTER 14

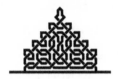

Ted: What Went Wrong?

I was compelled to dig deeper into why the first fusion had failed. I thought maybe it was just bad luck perhaps, but the device was doomed from the onset.

I later discovered this type of device pulled the healing process off to one side of the vertebrae. That, in itself, is why I didn't fuse on the other side of the spinous processes (or more specifically, to the bony projections off the back of the vertebra on that side) and that no matter what I did, it was going to be horrible every time I stood upright from then on.

Going through all my notes that I had recorded, I started to suspect that Dr. Clack omitted the extraction step of seeding the fusion (that is, from taking bone from my hip) during the surgery and relied solely on the bone growth stimulator to create the fusion. He did use some of the bone from the laminectomy, because that was going to happen anyway when he "routed out" the transforaminal canal to enlarge the opening of the nerves that pass through it. In any case, it seemed that Dr. Clack thought the little bit of bone along with the stimulator would likely be sufficient for fusion to occur. This small but important detail, however, he neglected to tell me both before and after surgery.

I believe Dr. Clack had to know that the bilateral fusion had not occurred on both sides of the L5-S1 vertebral area. I believe that Dr. Clack hoped that by leaving that battery in me, it would eventually cause the area where he had performed the surgery to fuse fully.

If it had worked the way it was supposed to, the new technique would have been revolutionary, and the use of this internally placed battery-powered bone growth stimulator would become the next generation of success by orthopedic surgeons all throughout the medically advanced countries of the world.

If Dr. Clack had discussed omitting the extraction step with me prior to surgery, would I have said, "Go ahead. I am young, healthy, and since you are using a secondary measure--the bone

Ben Dales and B. B. Beaudreaux

growth stimulator--we're guaranteed success"?

I just might have, who knows? Then again, maybe I would not have. The point is, I never had the opportunity to decide for myself. The device manufacturing company aggressively pushed this decision upon the doctor. The company cited statistics based solely upon (as I've since learned) its own "self peer review." This prevented an objective, real-life vantage point about its device.

I trusted Dr. Clack, as most everyone does with their surgeons; otherwise patients surely would not give their surgeons consent to operate.

The resulting problem in my case, however, was that the device did not work. And the little bit of bone from the "routing out" of the canal was not enough to bridge the gap between the two intended points of fusion.

To his credit, I believe Dr. Clack was actually trying to spare me the pain of extracting the bone from my hip and therein make it less painful for me to go through this surgery. Nevertheless, there is a degree of separation between me as the patient and him the surgeon, versus the promoters of the device that he was using for the fusion. He was simply going by what the company was telling him.

As it turned out, the fusion device was later pulled from company promotion and from the market. This was done covertly and quietly. There was no mention to any potential patients that events like mine, i.e., non-fusion results, were happening. I didn't know what was going on; I was not a doctor.

But Dr. Clack did know. When he was examining my X-rays, I recalled vividly how his face would become red. This was the clue to me that he was holding back some information.

"Why is my left leg in so much more pain than before the surgery, doctor?" I asked.

"I don't understand why you're in more pain as the X-rays appear to show that you have partially fused."

"Well, can't you re-rout out the canal more on the left side?"

"I did that," said Dr. Clack. "There should be plenty of space so that there is no bone impeding on the nerve root as it exits this level."

The truth was, the fusion on the left side was not solid--so every time I stood upright, or sat in an upright position, the canal on the left side would slightly close and press on that left nerve root. But this was not told to me by Dr. Clack.

Ben Dales and B. B. Beaudreaux

This is why Dr. Feisler determined I had to have the first surgery redone. This second surgery, however, was to be a lot more difficult in practice than theory. Sure, it would be easy enough to fuse the bones using a cage between the actual column--but first he was going to have to break apart the section of the vertebrae that did actually fuse. Orthopedic surgeons know that once a bone fuses, it will never break in the same place again because the "new" bone is of greater strength than the original bone.

Dr. Feisler was upfront with me about this.

Redo.

He told me the reason he was going to have to take apart the bone where it had fused was because otherwise he could not align the bone correctly, due to my mild case of Spondylolisthesis. When I asked him if he had ever done this particular surgery before, he truthfully told me that he had not, that this was a very complicated case now.

He went on to share that he did in fact know very well how to use a chisel and hammer, since one of his hobbies was furniture making.

A chisel and hammer?

CHAPTER 15

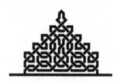

Deni: Thoughts Before Surgery

The hospital is somewhere way up north, actually in one of the city's northern suburbs.

Thinking back, the location was a minor concern, even if we would have to travel more than 30 miles one way to get there. The bigger concern is--how did we get to this point in the first place? Why is there going to be a second surgery?

I recalled the horror of the first surgery and its aftermath. It was a long wait during the surgery itself, sitting in that waiting room. I even remember my near panic as only an hour or so after Ted was wheeled off for his predicted four-hour surgery, there was an emergency situation in the surgery area with shouts of "Code Blue" and with many gowned hospital personnel rushing and running into the restricted surgery area. I was scared it was

Ted, but later found out it was another patient.

It was what brought us to this day, one which was directing us to some heretofore unknown location north of Chicago.

As we were driving northward that day, we were commenting on the fact that it's not even in the city, not like before when we were up on the north side at a well-known hospital facing Lake Shore Drive and viewing Lake Michigan. This time we had to find a remote (to us) location hospital in the northern suburb of Skokie. I had been to this suburb maybe twice in my life; I had not grown up in Chicago either, or even in Illinois. All that I truly knew or perceived about Skokie was that it existed as an affluent suburb mostly populated by Chicagoland's Jewish community, the most famous of which was one of our all-time favorites--Bette Midler. Not that she lived in the area anymore, as she of course had moved on to bigger and better.

But I digress. There was no fast-track route to get us to this hospital on the day of surgery. It was actually our first time ever there, since we had done our pre-surgery consultations with Dr. Feisler in his Chicago office, and we had completed the usual required pre-registration for the hospital over the phone. Although we didn't know this at the time, Dr. Feisler was entering into a professional partnership with Dr. Clack. This partnership would later be detrimental to us.

To say that we weren't apprehensive leading up to this surgery would be a lie. After all, we had been so extremely optimistic and hopeful about Ted's first surgery, only to have our dreams and hopes about it gradually and slowly crushed during the near past two years since it had happened.

This time, we were cautiously optimistic.

Ben Dales and B. B. Beaudreaux

CHAPTER 16

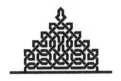

Ted: Surgery Day...Again

What am I doing here again?

I keep asking myself this same question.

I don't believe this. I was guaranteed the pain in my ankle and the recurring lower back strain would be fixed by the first fusion.

I'm praying this surgery will give me my life back.

I cannot accept I am in the hospital. Again. This time it's not because of anything I did, but because of what another doctor put inside me. And to top it off, it happened after I'd worked so hard and finally had obtained the greatest job--one where I could travel, use my language skills, and meet new people.

Yet, here I am again--over a year since Dr. Clack threw up his hands in the air and said, "I really don't understand it. To me it seems the bone growth stimulator worked fine on one side of the vertebral column. I can't understand why it did not work on the other side."

He was trying to blame it on my body's failure to heal properly--as opposed to something about the surgery itself. But the X-rays did not lie. The device did nothing to stimulate bone growth to promote the L5-S1 fusion.

If Dr. Clack had extracted bone from my posterior pelvic girdle (my hip), the fusion would have adhered to both sides. However, the device company's representatives told him he could omit this normal part of the fusion process by using their latest and greatest bone growth stimulator device. My own body simply did what it was supposed to do. It had fixed what it perceived as a broken bone on one side of my body.

Despite all of the unanswered questions, Dr. Clack could only muster a farewell handshake. There was nothing more he could do.

So I put my trust in Dr. Feisler. He seemed convinced he could repair the mistakes.

Ben Dales and B. B. Beaudreaux

What was Dr. Feisler thinking about when he knew he had to take apart the surgery of another doctor?

Had they spoken to each other about it?

I was hoping they had.

Why aren't they telling me the whole story?

I know why. It would scare the crap out of me!

But this surgery is my last chance. If I bolt from this room right now, no one will ever help me.

The nurse just came in again. At least this time, she was finding a vein in my arm instead of having to use my neck like last time.

She can tell I'm nervous. "This will help. It's going to be okay."

The sedative is kicking in. I'm trying not to think about the recovery.

I'll get back in the pool. Yes, the water...I'm gonna be back in the pool in no time.

Dr. Feisler assured me that I would get my mobility back.

I looked at the ceiling lights as they wheeled me down the hall into the operating room.

"It's cold in here. My arm is so cold." No one seemed to hear me.

Oh, please let this be an easy one, and even if it's not, just put me back the way I was.

The mask is preventing the tears from running down my cheek.

"I, oh, so hope..."

I was out.

In the Middle of Surgery

"...uhhhHHHHHHA AAHHHHHHHH! My leg hurts!"

"Can you feel this?" A voice asks.

"AGHHHHHHH! What did you do to me?"

"Can you feel it when I pinch your left leg here?" Dr. Feisler asks.

"AGGHAAHHHHHHH!!!!"

"You HAVE to tell me before I can close!" The same voice pleads. I feel a hand slapping me with force on my face. "Can you feel this?"

"AGHHHHHHH! Yes! Yes, I feel it bad!"

"What's bad?"

 Ben Dales and B. B. Beaudreaux

"IT HURTS SO BAD!!!!!!"

"What hurts?"

"My right leg. MY RIGHT LEG!!!"

"Can you feel the pinch on your right leg?"

"Yes. YES. AGHHH!!!" I don't recognize my own voice. It sounds like an animal screaming.

"Put him back out - NOW! NOW!"

I'm out again.

After the Surgery

"Oh, God! My legs are on fire!"

I see my neighbor Cora standing at the edge of the bed with Deni next to her. The surgery is over, but the pain is extremely intense.

"Calm down, Ted." Cora gently takes my hand. "Just calm down."

"Aghhhhhh!"

"Tell me, what do you see?" Cora asks. "Honey, what do you see in your mind?"

"I see...er, I see...aghhhHHH!" Waves of pain sweep over me again and again. "I SEE A MOUNTAIN! I see a man on a mountain. IT'S

JESUS! He's on a mountain...and the forest is below him. It's, it's, it's on FIRE!!! Aghhh! Look at Jesus!"

"Do you see him?" Cora asks quietly. "What is he doing?"

"He's crying. He can't stop crying. His mountain is burning--it's BURNING. The forest... it's a forest fire sweeping down the mountain. There's smoke. I smell smoke!"

"Okay. Listen to me. Listen to me! You're going to put out the fire," Cora commands gently, trying to soothe me. "You're just going to put it out now."

"I can't. It's too big, it's sweeping down on me."

"Just put it out." Her voice is sweet and calm.

"I can't. I can't!" I gnarl back.

"Then look away. Look the other direction."

"The fire is in every direction. The only other direction is up!" I screamed.

"Then go up. Just go up and away from the fire."

I notice Deni at the back of the bed, looking bewildered. Deni doesn't know what to do.

"Please, please. Help me. I'm suffering! The

window! Open it, please...let me jump!" I tried to reach for the window. I had to get away from the pain...and the fire.

"What is all this screaming going on in here?" The nurse in charge comes in. Her voice reminds me of Nurse Ratched from One Flew Over The Cuckoo's Nest.

"He's in pain," said Cora. "Give him something now!"

"Well, he just got out of surgery." Nurse Ratched counters.

"Give him more morphine now," Cora demands.

"Who are you?"

"I am Dr. Cora Lane. But it doesn't take a doctor to see that this man is suffering beyond words. Now go get his physician to increase the morphine drip before he has a stroke. And he will, if you do not do it." The loving, calm person has now reverted to her "Physician in Charge" demeanor.

The nurse hurries out the door.

"Look at me. Look at me, Ted! She will get you something, but it's going to take a few minutes. So you have to pay attention to my words," said Cora, the calm, collected, and loving nature returning to her voice. "Close your eyes and tell me about the mountain."

"It's still on fire."

"Then float above it. Just fly away from the fire."

"We're flying," I reply. "We're flying up over the mountain."

"Who's with you?"

"Jesus," I moaned. "I couldn't just leave him there."

"That's good, just keep away from the fire."

"I'm trying to stay away, but it's a big fire."

"But you're bigger than the fire, Ted. You can rise up over the fire. You just keep flying above the fire and look for water. Look for cool, cool, water…." Her arms were now moving energy out and away from my spinal trauma. "Do you see the cool water?"

"Not yet," I cry.

"It will find you."

"I hope the morphine finds me first."

Ben Dales and B. B. Beaudreaux

"Just keep floating away from the pain. In fact, you can't see the fire anymore, can you?"

"No, BUT I CAN FEEL IT...AGGGHHHHH!!!!!"

"Just keep floating above, flying away. Concentrate, Ted. Float away from it." Her arms were in full motion inches above my body.

"We're moving you away from the pain, and I'm moving all this junk away from you. Just concentrate on moving away, moving away."

"What have they done to me?" The tears flying from my eyes faster than the floating by me and Jesus above the mountain.

"Float away, just float away...."

CHAPTER 17

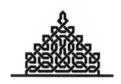

Deni: Surgery Day…Again

Father Jim, our good friend and the rector of our neighborhood church, insisted on being with us that morning. His "excuse" was that he believed someone needed to keep me company during the predicted six-hour surgery, but I believe it was also to give Ted as much spiritual assurance prior to going under the knife for the second time as he possibly could. He wanted Ted to take the Holy Spirit into the surgery with him.

Father Jim arrived early enough to be with us during the pre-surgery waiting period, and he and I stayed with Ted as long as we were allowed. Jim was intent on sending Ted into surgery with a prayer, which the three of us did together.

However, do not get me wrong. Father Jim was there for me every bit as much as he was for Ted, and I so truly appreciated his company during

Ben Dales and B. B. Beaudreaux

the first half of my waiting period. Naturally, as any busily-scheduled rector in Chicago, he told us in advance he would not be able to stay there the whole day as I (of course) would be doing. Therefore, we had requested and scheduled two other very good friends--Cora and Tyger--to come by during the early afternoon to finish the wait with me. Around noon when the first one, Tyger, arrived with food, Father Jim was able to excuse himself and depart for the day with a prayer and the promise he would return tomorrow.

The six-hour wait was underestimated. It was a full eight hours before we were notified of anything. It was an excruciating wait to say the least. Tyger's presence was a godsend, just as Father Jim's had been.

My first notification following surgery was supposed to be in person from Dr. Feisler. However, the surgery took two extra hours, and this doctor's need to go right into his next surgery prevented that. I had no clue that Ted was already in the recuperation area. After so many hours, this little message would have gone a long way.

Although I was very upset by this lapse of information supplied to us, departing the elevator I immediately began to experience a deja vu moment.

When I walked into Ted's hospital room after his first surgery two years prior, he was a vision of wires and tubes with the facial expression of someone looking many years older. I can still recall how pitiful he had looked to me, in every sense of the word. I began crying and could not stop. It took Ted at the time to calm me down; yes, he the patient had to console me. I wondered if this time it would be similar, as I gathered up my strength and emotions as best I could.

As we approached his room this time, we heard him before we saw him. He was moaning and screaming from the pain he was experiencing. Rather than divulge myself an emotional moment after entering the room, this time I immediately paged a nurse to help him. Ted told us amidst his moans that he had been given medication of some sort, but it wasn't helping. He was in terrible pain. He verbalized how all that he wanted right now was to die. He even asked if we could open the window for him to be able to jump and end it all.

Our other good friend Cora had arrived, and just in the nick of time. You see, in addition to being an ophthalmologist, Cora was a holistic healer... and a good one. She was also one of Ted's very, very best friends and former next door neighbor to us.

We entered the room, hearing Ted's screams. She looked at me and at our other friend standing there helpless to do anything more to quell the pain.

Cora took over and used some visualization techniques with Ted. It was not easy, but she somehow was able to capture his undivided attention. This was something I was unprepared to do, being filled with emotion myself.

It was unbelievable what Cora was able to do. She and Ted together took a "trip" led by his visualizations. Exact details escape me now. I was on an emotional edge just watching and hearing him scream in so much pain, but I do recall it involved a burning mountain and Jesus. She got him to think about something other than the pain (although I believe the "burning" part was an analogy for the pain he was feeling).

At some point, I'm not sure when, she lost him and he started screaming again loudly enough to be heard out in the hospital corridor. An unfriendly nurse came in and added to the screaming. Cora took over and demanded the nurse contact a doctor to get Ted some pain relief. Whatever Cora said, or probably how she said it, the nurse complied. Feeling so helpless myself, I was forever grateful at the time that Cora had taken charge.

While the nurse was gone, Cora went right back to work on visualization with Ted. She was so calming and reassuring that he followed her lead, at least until the nurse returned with more pain medication--additional morphine. It was a morphine drip that he was allowed to control. He gave it all he had, and once the morphine starting kicking in, it was obvious.

He eventually dozed off into slumber and, seemingly, pain relief.

Ben Dales and B. B. Beaudreaux

CHAPTER 18

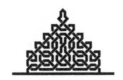

Ted: Recuperation from the Second Surgery

The days following the second surgery that crippled me are so very difficult to retell here.

This is not to say that they are difficult to remember vividly. It is, rather, the experience was so painful that it truly brings back the nightmare of what happened to me. Waking up after that second surgery was one of the most horrifying moments I have ever experienced.

Since the orthopedic surgeon, Dr. Feisler, felt that the vertebrae needed to be realigned, the only way to do that was to attach my body to a device that literally stretched me apart. This required the use of straps around my rib cage and torso and yet other straps around my waist, my hips, and my legs. My entire spinal column was stretched in an effort to get the metal instrumentation into the proper places for the vertebrae to fuse, and the nerves were stretched with them. It was the equivalent of being put on the rack and pulled apart--just like they did in the torture chambers of monstrous villains during the Middle Ages.

This contraption had been developed for use in people with curvature of the spine and the surgeries that children would face if they had that affliction. It truly was exactly the same as a medieval torture rack. I was told this procedure was the only way the orthopedic doctor could be sure he was pinning the rods, screws, cages, and aligning pins in the correct spot.

The problem that I faced as a 38 year-old man was that my nerves had grown to the length my body had already determined they should grow during puberty. Although it is possible for the nerves in one's spinal cord to be repositioned, special care must be observed when these nerves are stretched like rubber bands. In my case, there was hemorrhaging happening in and around the dura. This event in effect crippled me beyond any further repair, resulting in my hundreds of free-waving nerve endings clumping together and causing irreparable damage. They are stuck together like that forever, just as if one might cook a box of spaghetti without stirring and then try to put it back into the box.

Ben Dales and B. B. Beaudreaux

This was especially true in the spinal area known as the cauda equina (translated from Latin as the "horse's tail"). It is where the nerves exit the spinal processes and travel to the extremities to which they govern movement and feeling. The entire bundle of nerves at the L5 region of my back was now all matted together as if it had been dipped in mud.

So after the surgery, both of my legs were going to be in horrible pain for the rest of my life, not just my left one. There was nothing that could be done about it. In fact, Deni later told me that the doctor said I might not ever walk again. In retrospect, I am glad no one told me that at the time.

I spent eight days in the hospital in unbelievable agony. On the morning of the eighth day, I learned that I would be transferred to a rehabilitation facility. This decision had been made in order for me to "work with the therapists who would be able to assess where I was going to end up living on a long-term basis."

Living? In this much pain? For the rest of my life?

I could not even begin to think of living like this--the rest of my life. Every time I moved my legs, the pain was excruciating.

Alas, the truth came out. In reality, I had used up the allotted time allowable by my insurance to remain in the hospital following this particular surgery. However, my insurance would still be able to pay for me to be in other facilities.

I had a terrible feeling the "other facilities" would be the kind of institutions that no one who had a choice would ever want to step foot in (not that I could right now), much less live there.

However, not really knowing at the time what "other facilities" meant (but fearing they would be horrible), I started to bargain with the doctors. I wanted to go home. I expressed this to everyone during the meeting we were having to determine my placement--including the physician, the nurse, and the hospital therapist.

I told them I had been able to sit upright but had not been allowed to get out of bed. I asked if I could have a very sturdy walker to see if I might hoist myself using my arm strength to get out of bed. I figured this was going to be done later anyway, whether I could walk or not. With the help of two strong orderlies and a lot of groaning and grunting, I managed to get my feet on the floor and hold myself in an upright position with the walker.

"Well, that's great," the physician said. "But you'll never be able to move, so accommodations are being set up for you at a convalescent home."

My God, I'm 38 and I'm going to an old folks' home.

I couldn't bear the thought, so I mustered every bit of strength I had in my arms and slid one side of the walker forward, then the other side. With my upper body strength, I pulled myself forward. I did this a few times, even though I was in agony.

"Wow!" The therapist exclaimed. "You do have unusual upper body strength."

My bargaining banter and determination finally paid off. The doctor agreed that I could go home since there were no stairs, but only if two conditions were met.

The first condition was that a nurse and a physical therapist would be there every day for the next month. The second condition was that if anything happened, I was to return to the hospital immediately.

So with the help of the orderlies and a prescription for 160 milligrams of Oxycontin plus 15 milligrams of Oxycodone and a plethora of other neurological types of pain and other medications, I was allowed to return home.

Once I was home, hours seemed like years but the days methodically passed one by one. The nurses and physical therapists came every day and helped me learn how to get out of bed on my own and then into the bathroom just a few feet from my bedroom. I was encouraged by the nurse to use my walker as much as possible. I did try to do the therapy, but it was so very painful just doing the getting out of bed and into the bathroom part. For over a month, that is about as far as I could move except for a couple of wheelchair visits to my surgeon's office.

Meanwhile, the whole surgery aftermath and resulting condition required me to be on so much medication that I am surprised I did not vaporize into a coma. In the early days at home following my surgery, I was advised to take over 175 milligrams of Oxycontin daily plus a variety of other things that were supposed to numb my entire brain and body. During these days when a nurse was making the daily visits to my home, she would always change the bandages as well as try to get me out of bed and walking. Looking back, I guess I can say she was also making sure I woke up every day.

Deni was trying to do as much as possible, but for me there was absolutely no getting comfortable no matter what was done. The nurse made sure

Ben Dales and B. B. Beaudreaux

I had proper nutrition, but eating anything was just like eating gruel. Nothing had any taste and because I was on so much medication, nothing would pass through my gastrointestinal tract. The nurse started pumping me with laxatives, which eventually helped, even if it meant I was passing it all at once. This, however, caused so many other problems, including rashes and getting my sorry rear end to the toilet fifteen times an hour. Sleep was elusive at best, because I could not find a comfortable position.

Finally after six weeks of this and no infection having set in, I went back to the doctor. X-rays showed that everything was where the doctor intended. However, I was in so much more pain. The pain in both legs was, in fact, a thousand times worse than before I had any surgery at all.

The surgeon told me that because the bones were where they were when I was growing up, putting them now in their supposed "right" place pulled the cauda equina like a rubber band, and nothing could ever fix that. He was a bone doctor, so he put the bones where he thought they should be. The nerves were just pulled along the way, pulled in a manner that they were never meant to be pulled.

So now, no matter whatever else would happen, my legs were going to hurt, throb, and cramp for the rest of my life. They would hurt not from the outside in, but from the inside out. I was told that eventually since they were constantly cramping, they could cramp into a state of atrophy. The only thing the neurologist could suggest was to keep them moving to try to fend off the atrophy. The problem was, the more I moved them with physical therapy, the more they would hurt.

After the incision became healed up after a few months, I asked the doctor if I might get back in the swimming pool. My local park district pool was less than five minutes away, and it had a lift chair that would lower me into the pool. I knew that would take the pressure off my back. I had used it after the first surgery for almost two years in an effort to keep my legs from atrophying. Dr. Feisler though it was an excellent idea, especially when he learned about the lift that would hoist me in and out of the water. At the time this lift chair was used for just two people--for me at age 38 and for a man in his late 90s who had suffered numerous strokes.

Going to the pool became my ritual. The water felt good. I was able to stretch my arms and get the blood circulating throughout my body. Even so, it was still painful. I did keep it up and eventually was going six days a week. Getting to and from the pool became routine. After many months, I started actual swimming. Although my legs rather just flapped along for the ride, it did keep them moving. Every day after my time in the pool, I would need to rest for three hours in bed.

After about six months, I was determined not to be so dependent on the walker. I asked a friend if he would fashion me a rugged, secure, rubber-tipped, tall staff for me to use. Quite frankly, I was tired of struggling with the awkward and cumbersome four-legged walker that was often difficult to maneuver. I also didn't need the lift anymore, because I could use the handles of the wall steps to get myself in and out of the pool.

The lifeguards at the park district were the best. Though they had been here for years (since high school), now as college kids they were really dedicated to whomever loved the water. Since I had been their "customer" previously, they were more than willing to get me moving again. This is what I think saved me from becoming wheelchair-bound. The lifeguards kept encouraging me to use my arms to move myself through the water day after day, and slowly, my legs started moving too. They really cared about me and with that, gave me the inspiration to keep moving.

CHAPTER 19

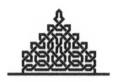

Ted: Reality Sets In

I was still on all those narcotics, so I really had no concept of how much pain I was actually experiencing until something preposterous arose that forced me to re-evaluate and adjust what I was taking.

Even though the cost of the medication was high, there was a more efficient alternative than going to the local pharmacy during the early 2000s. Mail-order bulk prescriptions were offered through my insurance in order to keep their costs down.

I decided to send in my prescriptions for mail-order processing shortly after I started getting in the pool (yes, Oxycontin was sent through the mail-order service back in those days). Because I was using a mail-order pharmacy to fill my prescriptions, I always made sure they were sent early--knowing the consequences of not having them would mean I'd have to return to the hospital.

Everything seemed to be going okay, as I continued sending my prescriptions to the mail-order pharmacists. They were sending me my orders on time until about five months into the process. I sent in my Oxycontin prescription, but the mail order service denied filling it. They stated that pre-authorization was required from the physician's office directly. The problem was that the service did not notify me there was going to be a delay. This was a preposterous happening in itself, but complicating matters was the fact that I learned this on a late Friday afternoon of a three-day holiday weekend.

I went into a bit of a panic.

Since I had only enough medication to get me through another day, I called the mail order service to see what could be done. I was led through a torrent of dead-end automated responses to trying to find out why I had not received my medication like I had before. When I finally reached an actual pharmacist, she demonstrated an attitude of "I'm in charge, and you're nothing but a damaged-goods low-life addict." She was not only uncaring and verbally abusive, but spoke to me in an extremely demeaning way. I tried to inform her that there was an urgency about the situation I would be facing with my needed prescription not having arrived by the weekend, but she interrupted with: "Well then, you shouldn't order the medication you depend on through mail-order," and--I swear to God--hung up on me with no resolution.

The only option left to me was to try to call back, which I did, only to get this very same woman who continued just hanging up on me. This happened a few times, as the automated system was not allowing me to reach any other person who would be able to assist me.

I called my doctor, but he was out of town for the holiday weekend, and I could not find another doctor that would prescribe me that type of very strong (C-II) medication without seeing me first. Instead, I was prescribed Vicodin, enough for five days until my mail-order prescription was supposed to arrive. I ran out of my regular medication on that Saturday and for the next five days I went from my previous daily 175 milligrams of narcotics to less than 35-40 milligrams of codeine.

The actual amount of pain I was really suffering from hit me like a brick wall. I did not have any withdrawal symptoms other than not sleeping--for some reason, I did not seem to be physically dependent on that type of medication. I remembered reading in a medical journal that some people just did not have the propensity to become

Ben Dales and B. B. Beaudreaux

easily addicted to certain types of medications as others did. However, lack of sleep was nothing compared to the pain I was forced to endure. This is when my true reality set in. I was going to be miserable for the rest of my life.

When the doctor finally returned from the holiday weekend, he rewrote the prescriptions but with a weaning schedule, because I was already off the large amounts of painkillers due to the mail-order screw-up. Even so, the major issue was that I was suffering miserably from the horrible pain. I continued to go to the pool, but the thought of living the rest of my life like this was more than daunting. It was like finding out I was the victim in a horror novel and that there was no way out.

To alleviate and compensate for the pain I was experiencing on reduced meds intake, the other medications were increased for me. These included Neurontin, Amitriptyline, and others. The Neurontin affected me (and others, I've since learned) horribly with side effects that include a disorienting feeling of uneasiness and anxiety. The Amitriptyline, which was increased to 100 milligrams, was explained to me as something that might help the pain even though pharmaceutical physicians could not really explain how or why it does work in "masking" the pain. The others prescribed were, like the Amitriptyline, used as a test toward circumventing the real pain I was going to suffer forever. All this was done in an attempt to find other means of controlling the pain. As it turned out, these attempts eventually proved futile.

The prospects of living in this crippled condition for the rest of my life made me question my very existence.

This is when my physical therapist suggested a service dog. I was hesitant, thinking I would not outlive the life of a dog--and that would be unfair to the dog. Just at that time, my friend Lon contacted me and told me his German shepherd, Sheba, was going to have puppies. Sheba was a wonderful dog. I had met her before any of these medical errors happened to me and knew her to be a caring, strong, and loyal dog. When Lon told me that puppies were on the way, I began thinking maybe a service dog would help me. To top it off, I had a very good friend who loved dogs and she told me that if anything happened to me, she would take care of any animal I had (including my two small furry cats that I had already rescued). So I made the decision and called Lon to tell him that I would like one of Sheba's puppies, and he told me I could have my pick of the litter when they were born.

Ben Dales and B. B. Beaudreaux

Thinking about having a dog lifted my spirits. I started really pushing myself to keep swimming though it was painful, and I had to lie in bed for hour upon hour when I was done. It was on one of my daily trips to the swimming pool that I found another furry friend.

I was dragging my tired self on my walk out of the recreation building to the parking lot when I saw a young mother with her two children in the park area having a picnic. They had a little black dog that reminded me of Toto from The Wizard of Oz. This dog, with one purple bow on her right ear, was unleashed and running back and forth around the park. I plodded over to where the young family was eating and told them that I thought their dog was cute, but that I was worried that it would run into the parking lot. The young woman told me that it was not their dog. She said it was hanging around them and that they had been throwing pieces of sandwich to try to get it to come closer to where they were eating in order to keep it out of the parking lot, but they were just about out of sandwiches. The kids could not get near the dog and neither could Mom.

I decided to go home but then thought of that little, frightened dog being hit by a car. Just knowing I could never rest with that knowledge, I grabbed one of the vegetarian bratwursts out of the fridge and went to the garage to get a large fishing net that I'd used when I was able-bodied and capable of going fishing as a hobby.

Grabbing that net made me recall for a second. I longed for my previous men's group of outdoor friends, with whom I would get out of the city and into the wilderness every once in a while for long weekend excursions year-round.

I returned to the park, and the dog was still there. I broke apart the sausage and threw a piece of it near the little black dog. The dog ate it immediately. The next one I threw a little closer to me. I was using the tall, sturdy staff while trying slowly to get myself into a position to maneuver the large fishing net, so I became motionless and did not scare the dog. She came closer with every piece of bratwurst I threw until finally she was in range of the net. I had only one chance, since I was unable to move quickly with my walker at the time, to try to catch the dog myself.

With one giant scoop I landed a "dogfish." Struggling through the net, I thought it was trying to escape, but the little black dog really only wanted the rest of the sausage, which she continued to eat through the net. I dragged the dog in the net the few feet back to the car and drove to the local veterinarian. I already knew the receptionists quite well, as we had developed a very close relationship over the years by my having brought in everything I had found and cared for, including turtles and even peacocks and peahens.

When I got there and explained my newest rescue, they chuckled and told me they would put out an APB about the dog. They also told me they were not able to keep the dog there, as all their kennels were in use at the time. When I told them I was in no shape to care for a dog, they said they could contact someone who would come over and pick it up. I took the dog home and put her in the basement, shut the door, and had to leave for an appointment with the neurologist on the north side of the city. I left a hurried note on the kitchen table for Deni, who at the time was teaching at the local high school (having transitioned out of the travel industry). BEWARE - DOG IN BASEMENT.

As for my neurologist's appointment, I was being sent once again back to the hospital to see Dr. Shep Allen. He was the neurologist who somehow convinced Dr. Feisler to take me on as a patient and try to fix the mess of the first surgery.

Dr. Allen was glad to see I was walking. He had known that the first surgery had failed and how traumatic the second surgery was going to be when he made arrangements for it with Dr. Feisler.

"How are you able to walk so well?" he asked.

I told him about my daily therapy in the swimming pool.

"That's good therapy. How are your pain levels?"

"Ever since the surgery, both of my legs are in severe pain all the time."

Evaluating this new slant to my problems, he insisted upon giving me another EMG (Electromyography) test.

"I want to see how badly damaged your nerves are in the area where your surgery was performed." As he explained it to me, he made sure to clarify that this test was not going to be fun.

"I remember having this test before, prior to my second surgery. In fact, you and Dr. Clack were the ones who required me to have it done."

"That's right," he acknowledged. "I remember now. Then you do know what it's all about."

Considering the amount of pain I was in, and since I trusted him as one who had previously gotten me to a surgeon that at least tried to fix what went wrong in the first surgery, we decided to take this step on the spot.

He left the room to retrieve a portable machine on a cart of its own. As I took off my trousers,

Ben Dales and B. B. Beaudreaux

he started by getting the machine set up for my EMG. The test itself was to begin with a series of shocks and increasing voltage amounts from a defibrillator type of device or paddles to several areas of my legs.

Once all was hooked up, my neurologist revved up the defibrillator paddles and shocked my legs three times in each muscle group (the calves, the thighs, and the hamstrings), each one with increasing voltage. Next, very thin needles three to four inches long were driven into the muscle tissue. This was in an effort to see if there are muscles firing indiscriminately due to nerve damage.

Having been through this before, I knew what to expect. What did bother me was knowing the needles that he was now going to insert deep into the muscle tissue would tell us what was going on. A still needle meant I was going to heal, or that there was little or no nerve damage. A jumping needle, along with a siren growing increasingly louder that emanated from an abnormality detected by the machine, meant there was severe damage which was permanent.

As he inserted the first needle, I could hear the audio on the detector go crazy. I was looking at the paper graph scrolling out the results as the test continued, and it was literally off the charts. I knew this meant my calf and thigh muscles were damaged beyond repair of my body's ability to heal.

"I need to test the hamstring muscle."

Dr. Allen inserted the needle into the back of my leg. This needle hit something that triggered my leg to pull the knee with a jerk back up against my hamstring and to cramp up into a locked position which I could not control.

He quickly pulled out the needle.

"Pull my leg down! **Pull my leg!**" I yelled.

Dr. Allen desperately tried to get my heel pulled back from its stuck position at the back of my hind end but could not muster the strength to do so.

I continued to yell. "Pull my leg down! PULL IT DOWN!"

"I can't! I can't get it to move!"

I flopped off the gurney and rolled myself around on the floor in such a way that I was able to stop the cramp in my muscles that had been holding my leg into this constricted position. The muscle finally relaxed. Dr. Allen had one hand on the top of my knee and the other was holding my ankle. The EMG machine toppled to the floor and wires were everywhere.

Ben Dales and B. B. Beaudreaux

It was a traumatic experience--for both of us.

I finally managed to straighten out my leg. We calmed down a bit, both of us still on the floor, he squatting and I just lying there.

"Wow, you have been able to keep your legs from atrophying with this swimming, haven't you?" Dr. Allen remarked after a beat of silence. "I would have never guessed you'd even be walking after what you went through."

He kept telling me to relax, but how could I? I was perspiring. Every graph reading was off the charts on every muscle group in my legs. Even Dr. Allen started sweating right along with me. I think it may have been hard for him to keep his physician's composure, because he was the one who had called in a favor with Dr. Feisler, whose attempted fix ended in disaster.

Could I put the blame on him? Absolutely not! He had already done what no other doctor would do. He used his connections in the world of medicine to find a surgeon who would take my case and try to fix another doctor's mistake because of the malfunctioning device that was pushed by a billion-dollar electronic device manufacturer. The surgeon he sent me to did the best possible job he could.

"Well, we most certainly got our answer."

I knew what he was saying. Once the nerves were damaged the way they were now, there was nothing more that could be done. I was going to be disabled for the rest of my life and suffer from horrible pain...forever.

Once we were finished with this test that admittedly almost finished both of us, Dr. Allen said, "It truly is a credit to you that you are walking after what you went through."

"I've always given everything my best, as I've told you, Dr. Allen, in everything I've faced in my life."

"Yes, I just saw that," he said, "and I have the readout of the EMG to prove that not only have you given it your best, but that the sad truth is this nerve damage is permanent. Your legs are going to hurt and cramp like this until they do atrophy. It's part of what's called muscular fasciculation. ALS patients have similar symptoms."

"Do you think I have ALS, Doctor?"

"No, no, absolutely not! That's one of the reasons I had you tested before with this EMG unit."

"Yes, I do recall when your associate Dr.

Nomaco did this very same test on me before the second surgery. She told me halfway through that she knew there was something wrong already, and decided to stop the test based on the readout she was getting for my left leg."

I told Dr. Allen how comforting it was that she had the empathy to stop the test right then, after observing the proof there was something wrong. She knew the primary probes proved there were fasciculations happening in my lower left leg, ankle, and foot. She knew there was no need to put me through the rest of this uncomfortable test.

"Dr. Nomaco is a very good neurologist, and she and I discussed your issue after the first EMG you had with her that demonstrated something was wrong after your first surgery," Dr. Allen replied. "She and I together convinced Dr. Feisler to try to fix that problem for you. Unfortunately, now you have what I can definitively rule as a disease caused by insult or trauma to the spinal cord. The disease is called 'Adhesive Arachnoiditis.' Have you ever heard of it?"

"No," I said. "Is it a rare condition?"

"Unfortunately, no, it's not rare for this to happen after surgery or certain types of injuries to the spine. The nerves that lead to your legs are all stuck to themselves in the center of the spinal cord, and they are also most likely adhered to the Arachnoid layer of the meninges. That is the very definition of 'Adhesive Arachnoiditis.' Additionally, there is the possibility of Cauda Equina Syndrome, meaning that nerves exiting your spinal cord at the bottom--where the cauda equina is--can be stuck together as well."

"You said 'meninges.' Is that as in meningitis?" I asked.

"Exactly. The meninges is one part of many in the human nervous system. It actually encases the brain and spinal cord."

"And Arachnoiditis, I know what that refers to," I said. "Arachnoid means 'spider.'"

"That's right, and that layer has blood vessels running through it that look like a spider's web, thus its naming convention." He paused for a few seconds. "You know, Ted, I think you should read a book called *Adhesive Arachnoiditis: The Silent Epidemic* by a very astute physician, Dr. Antonio Aldrete. It's a medical journal, so you'll really have to put on your thinking cap, but you have the smarts to understand what has happened to you. I hope you will read it."

Ben Dales and B. B. Beaudreaux

He continued on. "Ted, you are young. You're strong. You're a very determined man--you'll make your way. Things will just be more difficult now, but that does not mean you can't still have a full life. You'll have a disability, but if you keep swimming and keep trying, you'll make your way."

Dr. Allen told me he had a friend at the hospital, Dr. Dan Dandico, who was a pain management physician. He told me this physician would be able to dictate a course of treatment that might give me a semblance of my life back.

"He won't be able to fix the damage to your spinal cord, but at least he can help control the pain," said Dr. Allen. "And hopefully the spasms in your legs like the one that just happened in this test."

We both looked over at the EMG machine, wires still awry.

"Man, you really had my heart pumping," he said. "I'm sorry to have put you through that, but it was the only way to know for sure if there is irreparable damage to your spinal cord."

"No, no, I understand," I said. "I just wish I didn't hear the word 'irreparable' come out of your mouth."

"Look at how far you have come. I would've expected most people in your condition to be rolling in here after what you went through, and here you are walking. You have to be the most determined patient I've ever had the privilege to work with. You have to keep trying. I know you'll keep trying."

"Thanks, Dr. Allen. Encouragement coming from you means the world to me."

"You're welcome, Ted. And stay in that pool no matter what, okay?"

Back home, I knew I had to tell Deni what happened. I could not come to grips with the fact that I was permanently disabled, so how could I relay it to anyone else?

I just wanted to go to sleep...forever.

I woke up when Deni arrived home from work.

"Hi, Honey. It looks as if you had a rough day. How did the meeting with Dr. Allen go?"

"Not well. We had an incident while he was administering the EMG test," I said.

"What happened? Are you all right?"

"What happened was that when he was administering the test, my hamstring cramped up

Ben Dales and B. B. Beaudreaux

with such force that Dr. Allen was unable to pull my leg out of it. I fell off the exam table and onto the floor. My heel was literally pulled back up to my hamstring muscle in a locked position and it was extremely painful."

"Oh my gosh. Did you get hurt?"

"Well, I rolled around on the floor until I was able to get most of my weight into a position where I was able to force the leg back open. I scared the crap out of Dr. Allen."

"Well, what did he say?"

"Deni....He said……..he said......"

I choked back the tears. Telling Deni was going to be harder than I thought.

I finally managed to get it out. "Dr. Allen told me that I am permanently disabled and that not only will I be in pain for the rest of my life, but that my legs will eventually atrophy."

"Oh, Honey. I don't even know what to say. I'm, I'm……..so sorry. Really, I am so sorry." Deni wrapped me in a hug.

Regaining my composure, I went into more detail about almost everything that transpired that day. It was a heartbreaking conversation. When I was finished explaining, we both just looked intensely into each other's eyes for what seemed like an eternity.

Then we heard a bark.

"Oh my God, I forgot about the dog in the basement."

With a bewildered look, Deni turned to me. "Dog?"

I looked at the kitchen table. My note was still there, untouched and unseen by Deni. Forgetting about my problems for a second, I opened the door to the basement where I had put the pup before I left for the doctor. It was a good thing--I mean, forgetting about the fact I was disabled. As I peeked in, I thought:

Now, what am I going to do with you?

Ben Dales and B. B. Beaudreaux

CHAPTER 20

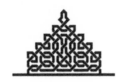

Deni: The Hard Truth

Shortly after Ted brought this rescued little dog home, we tried to locate its owner by going to the local vet's office to inform them of our found dog. We also posted notices at the park district fieldhouse on whose property we found her. There were no responses, and meanwhile this little dog captured our bleeding hearts, of course. Even though we had already agreed to take the pick of the litter from our friend Lon, which would give us another dog just a few months later, we could not help but keep this little dog.

So, we were about to go from a home with no dogs and two cats to one with two dogs and two cats. Nevertheless, we proceeded to name her, which naturally would seal our decision to keep her. The name choice came from Ted's favorite film, Elvira: Mistress of the Dark. In the movie, Elvira inherits a properly-coiffed toy poodle from what appeared to be her prim and proper deceased aunt. The poodle's name is "Algonquin." Elvira immediately gives the poodle a punk rock-groomed haircut and names it "Gonq." Thus, our new toy poodle became Algonquin with the preferred nickname of "Gonq." This dog became the love of our life. The unconditional love and companionship provided by Gonq and our other pets gave both of us much-needed loving assistance in dealing with the tragedy to befall our lives.

After Ted told me his grim prognosis, I could not take it all in, at least at the start, that Ted's situation was going to be permanent. I heard the words, but they could not totally register for me.

I had always been an optimist at heart, always adhering to the old adage of my favorite baseball team that "Hope Springs Eternal." I was unable to give up hope completely that something more could be done.

Probably more than anything, I finally had to let go of my hopes by listening to the reactions of others we told about the hopeless prognosis. I still recall distinctly when we told one of Ted's closest relatives (and who was by now also close to me) about the news. Rather than express sorrow and empathy immediately to Ted, this relative right away looked at me and said, "You're screwed."

Ben Dales and B. B. Beaudreaux

This comment, as I dwelled upon it, hit me squarely in the face and in the heart. I had to accept facts. I had to figure out how we were going to live with this.

My role as a caregiver was going to be a permanent one.

CHAPTER 21

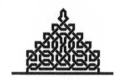

Ted: What Led to the Next Surgery

After a week or so had passed, I was set up with an appointment to meet the new pain management physician referred to me by Dr. Allen. To say the least, I was extremely unhappy to learn from Dr. Allen that there was irreparable damage to my spinal column. I was upset that even though the second surgery may have solved the fusion problem, it left me in a worse condition neurologically, worse than before I went under for the second time, and worse overall than when this entire fiasco began.

This pain management physician seemed to be the only recourse left for me.

I quickly learned that Dr. Dan Dandico was very passionate about his duties as a pain management physician. He demonstrated extreme interest in

Ben Dales and B. B. Beaudreaux

my relating all that transpired prior my coming to him as a patient. He questioned me about what brought me to the first surgery.

"I had been a healthy athlete," I told him. "I was a competitive volleyball player. This all started when I was experiencing pain in my lower left leg and left ankle."

I went into all the details that followed my life and about how I ended up having a second surgery to fix the first one. I told him how neither worked as they were supposed to have worked and that the pain was now in both of my legs, due to what Dr. Allen had referred to as Adhesive Arachnoiditis. I also told him Dr. Allen wanted me to read a book by Dr. Antonio Aldrete called *Adhesive Arachnoiditis: The Silent Epidemic*.

"Dr. Aldrete?" He questioned. "Well, I know him personally. We have attended conferences together. He is a very intelligent man. And you say that Dr. Allen wants you to read his book on Arachnoiditis?"

"Yes, he does."

"Then Dr. Allen must think you are a pretty smart guy. That is a highly technical book written mainly for physicians who have come across this issue in many patients like yourself, who have had poor outcomes with surgeries."

"Well," I chuckled, "I do have highly technical skills, although not in medicine--in computer operating systems."

"Ah, so you're a techy. Well, I tell you what, Ted. I will call Dr. Aldrete. As a matter of fact, I will call him right now, so we can get that book to you right away."

At that very first appointment, he was on the phone with Dr. Aldrete's office.

"Antonio! How are you? This is Dan, Dan Dandico from Chicago. How are things down in Florida?"

I could hear some response in the background over the phone.

"Good, good. Hey, listen, I have an extremely bright patient in my office right now who wants to read your book, *The Silent Epidemic*."

"No, he's not a medical student, he's my patient."

"Yes, but he has had issues with surgeries and already I am sure he is more than capable of understanding."

Ben Dales and B. B. Beaudreaux

"Yes, I think it will definitely help him understand what is going on with his condition."

"Sure. His first name is Ted and yes, that would be great. Send it to me at the hospital here in Chicago…yes, that's right. Uh huh, yes, I'll make sure he gets it. No, write it to him, yes, write it out to his name Ted."

I was quite impressed that my new physician would call this other physician and author with me in the room--on the fly--just like that. He had the confidence to, out of the blue, talk to the most leading researcher in the world who wrote about the disease I was suffering from and actually order the book for me.

"Well, you're going to have some homework to do, Ted. It will require you to do even more research on the human nervous system. Think you can handle it?"

"Yes, I want to know what's going on more than anyone," I replied.

"Now let's go through your list of medications you are currently taking."

"Sure." I opened my medical journal. "I've written everything down in here."

"Wow, you have your own medical journal?

May I see that?" With a downward tilt of his forehead, looking over the top of the journal I just handed him, he said, "You know, you're the only patient I've ever seen with an actual personal medical journal."

"I think everyone should keep one! Do you know how hard it would be to keep track of all that has happened to me without this?"

Dr. Dandico and I spent almost an hour together in this first appointment. After he took careful notes on all the medications I was taking, he asked me what I was doing for physical therapy. Of course, the details about every day in the swimming pool was the main topic.

"Great, so you are using your legs in the water too?"

"Well, yes, but I'm not pushing it. I could barely use my legs after the second surgery, so I used my upper body to propel me through the water. Over time, I started being able to use them gently to provide a little thrust through the water. If I overdo it, they cramp up--especially afterwards."

"Okay then, we need to give you something to control those cramps in your legs. You know what those cramps are called?" He asked.

"Yes, they are muscular fasciculations, and they are caused by damaged nerves within the spinal column as they exit the foraminal canal. The damaged nerves causes the muscles they control to fire from deep within the muscle tissue as if the brain were telling them to move."

"Hey, you do know your stuff," he excitedly replied.

I could tell Dr. Dandico was really happy when he was talking to patients who took interest in what was happening to them in regards to their own health. It was at that moment that I realized that he was not the old-guard type of physician, and that he wanted people to manage their own health issues--because after all, it was their lives on the line.

"Dr. Allen and I had, well, an 'incident' during my last EMG test. It was then that he explained what my test results were and why they were abnormal by explaining about fasciculations."

"Then he taught you how to read the graph results?"

"Didn't have to," I grimaced. "My hamstring cramped up so horribly while he was administering the test that it literally knocked me off the table and onto the floor. I could hear the audio on the machine going nuts prior to that happening, so I knew something was wrong."

"Plus," I continued, "I had that very same test procedure before with abnormal results, so I kind of figured that the results were going to read that there was something definitely wrong. I felt the results were going to confirm my suspicion that now there was a consistent and permanent injury not just in my left leg, but in both legs."

"Knocked you right off the table, eh? What did Shep--I mean, Dr. Allen, do?"

"He just tried to help me straighten my leg out, but I think that incident gave him a bit of a fright."

"So what do you think might help control these fasciculations?"

"Well, since the muscles are contracting, I suppose we would want to use some type of muscle relaxer?" I guessed.

"Yes, good. Have you ever used them before?"

"No."

"No, huh? Well, what type do you think would be useful without causing too many side effects?"

"I'm guessing one of the benzoids, maybe Valium?"

Ben Dales and B. B. Beaudreaux

"Correct! The most frequently used one is Valium or Diazepam. Let's try five, maybe ten milligrams at bedtime," he suggested. "Keep a log and report back if you see a change. Now, what about other meds you are currently being prescribed?"

"Well, for the pain, Norco, two to three times a day."

"Do you know what that is?"

"Yes, it's Tylenol, or acetaminophen with codeine."

"Exactly. Is it effective?" He asked.

"I'm getting by, but I'm never not in a high level of pain," I admitted.

"And how long have you been on Norco, or even Vicodin?"

"Since my first surgery. That was to address the pain I was experiencing just in my left leg and occasionally in my lower back."

"Have you had blood work done to check your liver functions?"

"Not recently."

"We better run a panel. And...do you drink alcohol?"

"No, that's the last thing I'd want to do with all that's going on is drink any alcohol."

"Ted, you know that it's not advisable for you to be on acetaminophen for long periods of time, right?"

"Yes, I did read that there have been some issues related to heavy usage of acetaminophen over long periods of time causing liver damage," I said, "but no one has ever offered me anything to use except those two medications. To tell you the truth, taking those pills always makes me a little nauseous."

"Okay, I've got an idea. Have you ever heard of Dilauded?"

"No."

"It's similar to how codeine works only there is no acetaminophen in it, and therefore it's less dangerous over long periods of time. Let's get you started on that. I'll prescribe four milligrams four times a day, but only take them if you need them. Understand?"

"Yes, I do. Also, I do need to tell you that

sometimes, if I forget to take my pill or if I'm in the pool a little too long, I have no choice but to get into bed and stay there for the rest of the day. That's why I'm always trying to be very systematic about when I need to do anything or go anywhere. It's frightening at times."

"Okay, let's see what else we can think of."

So on and on we went until I had about five different prescriptions in my hand. Only two were controlled, all with very explicit instructions on how, when, and when not to take the medications he was prescribing. He wanted me to call him back in a week, or immediately if I had any issues with the prescriptions. As he talked, I was writing all he was saying in my journal.

What he told me was this: "Ted, if you have any, and I mean any, issues with these medications, call me immediately. Understand?"

"Okay, I will, but I don't want to have you paged after hours. I mean, I know you have a personal life too."

"No, no--I'm giving you my cell number. You call me directly if you have any issues or questions with any health concern."

"Really?"

"Yes, you can call the office first during working hours if it's not an emergency, but if you need to get in touch with me after hours, here is my cell number and my personal email address."

This had been the first physician I had ever seen, or as he wanted it phrased, "worked with," who was willing to give out his email address and direct cell number. He was so different than any other physician I ever had before.

So this began not only a doctor-to-patient relationship, but also a person-to-person relationship which lasted years. As we worked out a pain management schedule together, we would try different things based on what would make my life "as manageable as possible."

I never needed to call him directly. I kept extensive notes in my journal, which I continued to bring to every appointment.

CHAPTER 22

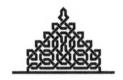

Ted: Trusting the Medical Profession

Dr. Dandico suggested, and I agreed to try, many different types of pain medications over the years I spent with him as my pain management physician. I continued to rely on his advice as the "best" and most "trusted" solutions to keeping me at a level of pain which I was able to tolerate.

As his career advanced and he accepted position at other hospitals, I always followed him. We had such a good rapport that no matter in what hospital he landed, I was going to follow him. He genuinely seemed to understand the issues I was facing on a daily basis and knew that mine was not a condition that I could heal from or that could ever get better. I never went to any other physician or clinics in an effort to garner other medications, because I knew he trusted me as I had been absolutely honest with him from the first day I met him.

Our doctor-patient relationship became stronger as the years passed. He trusted me, and I trusted him with anything that he might suggest or at least ask me to consider. I too would do as much research as I could on the internet or by reading books about human neuroanatomy and about any new treatment or medication that might be in the development stages. He likewise would find out about different treatments or medications that were "new" on the market to alleviate the complication of severe pain I had from the first two surgeries. Of course he had a plethora of knowledge about all the newest pain medications and treatments being offered to those in need, because pharmaceutical and other entities who were in the business of pain management would solicit him since he was an anesthesiologist.

When the "patch" was first produced to control pain transdermally (through the skin), he suggested that I give it a try. This is when my medication was changed from 6 "pills" a day to 1 "patch" every three days.

This medication, which adhered to the skin and delivered the dosage transdermally, was Fentanyl. The Fentanyl patch worked extremely well to control pain--on the first day, but the amount

Ben Dales and B. B. Beaudreaux

of medication it delivered to the body depleted precipitously when a single patch was supposed to last three days. The issue I faced, was that by the third day, I again was in horrible pain. So he adjusted me to a very specific regiment. One which did control the pain.

This regiment was:

On the first day of a three-day run, I was to apply a 50-microgram patch. The third day I was to put on a 12-microgram patch, and then the fourth day I was to remove both patches and start all over again with a new 50. This was an extremely powerful pain medication and the ups and downs affected me severely after being on this cycle for about a year. It was during that year of this medication regimen when I reported to him the major "side effect" of this medication. This was because, as I found out while using it, this medication affected my sleeping rhythm. This specific "side effect" was not listed on the accompanying literature that came with this medication. For me, my normal sleep pattern was completely interrupted. For the first 24 hours after I attached the 50-microgram patch to the skin, I found sleep elusive. Then, the next two days, I would be extremely tired all the time.

We mutually decided to remedy this "side effect" with the use of a medication called Provigil.

I would take this on the second morning after I adhered the 50-microgram patch. It did work to keep me awake and alert the second day, but soon it got to the point where I was a walking zombie. Even though it was extremely effective in controlling pain, I asked him to take me off this regimen and put me back on what I was taking before. This was so I could control the dosage better even though it was less effective at controlling the pain overall.

As Dr. Dandico's career continued to evolve, so too did our relationship. When he left the hospital where I first met him for another opportunity in the west suburban area of Chicago, I followed him to that hospital.

Dr. Dandico was also fluent in Spanish. At times we would throw a phrase in Spanish at each other to see if both of us were paying attention regardless of the language being spoken. I recall that one word we threw around within an idiomatic phrase was the Spanish word tortuga, which means "turtle" or "tortoise." This all started from a conversation we had about how Deni and I had won a free trip to the Galapagos Islands far off the Pacific coast of Ecuador. I used the trip as an opportunity to study botany there, but had become fascinated with the giant turtles called tortoises. Dr. Dandico acquainted this story into a Spanish language analogy about my ongoing pain and how we were treating it. He made the comparison in Spanish to Aesop's Fable of "The Tortoise and The Hare" and the idiomatic conclusion that "Slow and steady wins the race!" From that point on, the word tortuga in our office conversations took on special meaning, such as how we might beat my affliction slowly and steadily.

I read the entire book sent to me by Dr. Aldrete, and although it was very, very medically technical, I gained a tremendous amount of insight on the Adhesive Arachnoiditis disease. Soon I found myself on different websites devoted to those of us dealing with pain issues, many of whom had no idea how insidious this particular disease truly was. Other websites shared how people were developing this condition after surgery, then only to be told by their surgeons, "Well, we have to go in again to try to fix what you are experiencing."

The truth was that for numerous persons who were suffering from Adhesive Arachnoiditis, no matter how many times they would have surgery, the pain was never going to subside. In fact, the more surgery they would have, the worse the pain would become.

Dr. Dandico and I discussed how Dr. Aldrete had written about neurosurgeons who tried to go in to the spinal column with extremely tiny instruments to try to separate the nerves that had been clumped together, or were stuck to the meninges. However, no matter how delicate or how precise the neurosurgeon was, the surgeries were futile. There is a good reason why this is true. Regardless of where the exact site of the "adhesions" or trauma is located within the human nervous system, all subsequent surgeries would result in even more scar tissue building up and thus more adhesions of the nerves to themselves and/or to the meninges.

After a number of years at the west suburban hospital, Dr. Dandico was offered the prestigious position as chief anesthesiologist at another reputable hospital in Chicago. Having such high regard for this doctor--who seemed genuinely concerned about and dedicated to me along with the rest of his patients--again, I followed him to his new hospital and his career as head of the department.

Often I could hear him through the corridors, while waiting to see him at his new offices, talking to patients whose native language was Spanish. He could not only understand but would converse with fluency that matched that of these native speakers.

His office had framed documents of awards that rated him "The Most Compassionate Physician of

Ben Dales and B. B. Beaudreaux

the Year" for three years running. He was the Chief of Anesthesiology and Pain Management. His staff members were top-notch. The administration team were all "on the ball," and things in his office always ran smoothly. He simply would have it no other way.

Dr. Dandico was keeping my pain level to a manageable level, one which was so important to maintain accurately. The reason why he did this was because the medications were opiates. And although I was at a low enough level that I could stop taking them without severe withdrawal symptoms, he was making sure I would not reach the level considered to be abusive.

Therefore, every few months I had to submit to a urine test to see if there were any illicit drugs in my system which he had not prescribed. I had no issues with this whatsoever, because I would never have thought of abusing the medications that were truly keeping me going. There was a further reason that the pain was kept at the threshold of a manageable level; Dr. Dandico also knew that the very medications that were working for me now would eventually need to be increased. We discussed how the mammalian body, when subjected to opiate medications in order to alleviate severe pain levels, systematically tends to build up a tolerance to those very medications.

So for years we maintained my pain medications at a low level, which allowed me to be able to continue with my swimming and other things too. But I was never allowed to return back to work. I had not received a note from any doctor stating I would be cleared to do so. Further, if I did so on my own, my disability insurance--upon which I relied--would be cut off. At first I really did think I might be able to work from home in bed. When the continuing and even increasing pain rendered that impossible, I slowly began to accept that my life would never return to "normal."

I was reading a lot, and one of the books I read was *Frida* by Hayden Herrera. This biography of Frida Kahlo disclosed how the late great artist had been in a street car accident that caused what would have been categorically described, with today's understanding of human neuroanatomy and of related diseases, as Adhesive Arachnoiditis. Yet, the author additionally reveals how Frida, with the use of small doses of opiates prescribed by her physician and similar to the ones I was now taking, became a world-renowned artist.

Inspired by the story of Frida, I started to paint. I was painting from my bed, just as Frida had done (except for the mirror on the ceiling). I had also found portable recliners that, although not as comfortable as lying completely flat, allowed me

Ben Dales and B. B. Beaudreaux

to get in and out easily enough to where I could access my paints, brushes, and canvases to create what I was told were beautiful works of art.

This was also when my friend Lon with the German shepherd gave me the pick of the one and only litter of puppies for his dog, Sheba. I picked the one I thought was the smartest in the bunch, because she cleverly escaped the pen while the others were stuck. I named her Heidi. Because she was so smart, house training her at eight weeks old took less than a day. She closely followed around my toy poodle Algonquin, or Gonq, and learned from her.

As Heidi grew into a juvenile puppy, she soon started to learn how to become my personal assistant and to do things that little Gonq could never do, being so tiny. If I dropped one of my paint brushes, even the most slender or narrow, Heidi would pick it up and hand it back to me. She would bring in the firewood. She would delicately pick up my glasses or keys if I dropped them. She would attentively sit at my side and watch for hand signals directing her to lie down or to sit or to go to the other room without my ever having to interrupt a conversation. Things began to seem like they might become manageable again.

Overall, I was starting to feel my life was somewhat workable again through Dr. Dandico's regimented pain management system. He seemed to be truly interested in not just managing my pain, but managing my pain while trying to have me lead as much of a "normal" life as I could.

And that is why I trusted him with anything he might suggest I try. Of course I had to, because anything that might help to alleviate the pain that I knew would be with me throughout the rest of my life was the only choice I had.

Dr. Dandico trusted me, but more importantly--I trusted him. I can honestly say, without a hint of doubt, I completely trusted him with my life.

CHAPTER 23

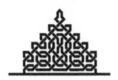

Ted: Six Years Later - Decision to Implant

"What company is it?"

Dr. Dandico showed me the brochure for the device with the manufacturing company's name, SAN Medical Device Company.

"I am not familiar with that company name nor have I ever heard of the device." I opened the brochure. "I guess if you say it could cut the amount of pain medication I am taking, I should be interested, huh?"

"SAN Medical makes many medical devices, and this is one of them," he explained. "It's called the Eon mini-neurostimulator."

"Well, what exactly does it do?"

"This is a device that interrupts pain signals coming from the base of the spinal column, so you will feel less pain."

"Have you had other patients who used these devices?"

"Yes, some patients say they've reduced their pain medication significantly," the doctor said. "The manufacturer just redesigned the new recharge unit with a new type of battery, so it's smaller and easier to implant."

"Well, I'd do anything to help control the pain."

"I'll have the company representatives come in, and we'll schedule you to meet them."

About a week later I met the first representative, Galli Vincenti. He seemed very pleasant and was very excited to promote the virtues of the "new and improved" mini-neurostimulator. He shared that this new device was the latest and greatest thing in controlling pain. He told me he had someone with personal experience who would tout the wonders of this device. The gentleman happened to live in Hawaii.

"This man can tell you all about it and how it cut the amount of pain medication he was taking," said Mr. Vincenti.

So I waited until that evening when, with the time difference, the call would be at a decent hour for the Hawaiian. When I reached this man by phone, he was approachable and cordial enough. The only problem was that he would not tell me the amount of pain medication he was actually taking. As it turned out, I learned later he was taking about ten times more medication than I had been, but I had no way to know this for two reasons. First, he wouldn't tell me. Second, his medical information was privately protected.

If he had been willing to tell me, I would have known that he was still taking more pain medication than I was--even though he already had the neurostimulator implanted in his back! What I did get from the conversation was that he hoped to have yet another surgery to have the newest, smaller mini-neurostimulator implanted in place of the larger unit he had in his back.

When I later talked to the office of Dr. Dandico, and consented to the idea of this implant, the staff had already been in contact with the SAN representative to get all my paperwork in order.

First, I would have a test unit implanted in my back, with wire leads dangling from behind me with a control module that I could use to turn the device on and off. The letters of approval promptly arrived in the mail and the test "surgery" was quickly set up. I was sedated for this implant, but afterwards I was sent home to try out the device.

The testing of this device was hard for me to gauge. The reason was because two small incisions had been made where the metal leads were going to be placed next to my dura. The rods that were inserted did hurt, and so did the incision. And of course I was on pain medication for the pain in my legs so it lessened the pain at the surgical site. Two wires dangled from my back at the base of those rods, and those wires connected to a power unit that I could control with a test unit. With this unit, I could send "shock waves" to those metal rods, which were supposed to act as a pain inhibitor. The theory was that these electric waves would interrupt the pain signals coming from my legs, which was constant. SAN had done testing on animals where they concluded that electric shock waves would lessen or interrupt the pain emanating from the damaged nerves in the spinal cord, which controlled motor function in one's legs. Or at least, that was what they were telling prospective patients like me who suffered permanent nerve damage from previous failed surgeries, or surgeries where mistakes had been made.

As I was making my way into the examination room at Dr. Dandico's office, I was thinking about

Ben Dales and B. B. Beaudreaux

how this had been such a hasty test for such a tremendously important decision to be made as to whether this electronic device would help alleviate the never-ending pain emanating from my legs. The problem with the test was two-fold. First, I was already on pain medication and there was no dictation from my surgeon to try and decrease what I was taking. And second, in order to implant the electric rods in my back, they had to make painful incisions that made it difficult to judge whether there was any effect on the pain emanating from my legs.

"Did it help with the pain?" Dr. Dandico asked me when I reported back with the results of my experience.

"Well, it is similar to a *TENS unit," I replied.

"Do you think it was a success?"

"I don't really know, since it was in me such a short time," I admitted. "The pain from the incisions made it so that I was forced to increase the amount of pain medication I had to take. So, there was really no way for me to gauge whether it made a difference."

Thinking back now, I realize I was really not in a condition to make such a decision.

"Just remember," said Dr. Dandico, "if after we

install it and it does not work, we can always take it out."

At the time I asked both the doctor and the SAN device representative, "How hard will the battery pack be to install?"

"It's so much smaller than all the previous models. It will be an easy procedure," the representative replied.

There I was, stuck with no alternative available to stop the pain. If I did not give this a try, I would never really know if it was the solution I so desperately sought.

So I said, "I guess it is a go."

But there was so much more for me to understand about having an electronic device implanted in my body. The test was not a long enough or sufficient way for me to gauge whether or not this "test" would be a way to control the pain emanating from my legs. It was too fast. It was too short. But most importantly, I did not have the whole unit implanted in the test. Yes, there was another component that would be installed after this test was completed. This additional component was a battery that needed to be recharged through my skin implanted in my hip. I had no idea the rechargeable battery was going to be the latest technology in power-storing devices--a lithium-ion battery.

The real truth was, I was grasping at anything that might help reduce the pain in my once strong and powerful legs.

*TENS: Transcutaneous Electric Nerve Stimulation

CHAPTER 24

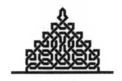

Ted: After the Implant Surgery

And so...it happened.

The "permanent" implant of the mini-neurostimulator was surgically placed into the thoracic region of my spine, accompanied by a rechargeable battery pack that was subcutaneously implanted in my hip.

Following the implant, I asked my surgeon, "Should I begin using it right away?"

He said yes.

A battery reading from a remote control revealed that the battery was not fully charged. I read the instructions and recharged it accordingly. I noticed my skin felt warm during recharging, but I had no reason to suspect this was anything but normal.

Later, I asked Deni to change the bandages.

"Oh, my God!" Deni stepped back in horror.

"What's wrong?"

"You have to look at this in the mirror."

Concerned, I got up from my bed to see what was going on. What I saw in the mirror horrified me, too. Deep purple bruises covered both incision sites.

"Take a picture, I need to send this to Dr. Dandico."

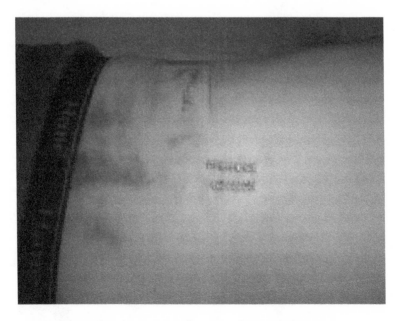

Photo taken by Deni and sent to the implant surgeon,
Dr. Dandico

The next thing we knew, I became seriously ill. I developed such a severe respiratory infection following my surgery that I had to be taken to the emergency room of a neighboring hospital. The ER was filthy--there was medical debris everywhere. Bloodied bandages that had yet to be thrown away sat on a nearby gurney with used gowns piled in a corner.

The bruising, combined with the fierce infection, prompted the on-call doctor literally to ask me if I wanted to stay in the hospital to battle the infection or "succumb" to it at home.

It was vastly unsettling, to say the least.

The ER staff told me they were going to report my condition to Dr. Dandico at the hospital where the implant surgery had taken place. Despite the pictures I sent and my admittance to the ER, no action was voiced or taken to address my concerns.

Was this was really just a normal part of the implant process? Look at the photos in this chapter and gauge your initial reaction to them!

Well, as you might guess and as it turned out, of course it was not normal.

Back to the episode of the emergency room visit, I made the decision to return home rather than be admitted. I was given a prescription for

Ben Dales and B. B. Beaudreaux

heavy-duty antibiotics and the send-off wish that I should just be as content as I could be while trying to "hang on."

I went home in extreme pain. For the first time since the second surgery when my spine was chiseled apart and then replaced with rods and screws and cages to put it back together, I reached way back into the medicine cabinet and took out the Oxycontin--medication I had been abruptly weaned off of since about six months after the reconstructive surgery.

At this point, to me, it did not matter. I remember taking 40 milligrams once, and then another 40 milligrams about 18-24 hours later while keeping the unused bottle of powerful medication from the reconstructive surgery away from my bedside. Even though I had that medication in the medicine chest, I never took it, except for this one incident after I was told not to by Dr. Feisler, the surgeon who tried to reconstruct what went wrong in the first surgery.

After that, I don't recall much about the next three days other than what was told to me by Deni later on. In and out of consciousness, I was forced to again take the antibiotics and pain medication that I had been taking prior to this latest surgery.

When I finally came out of my infection-induced mode, Deni had contacted Dr. Dandico and told me an appointment was made for me to see him the following week.

At the appointment, the doctor greeted me as if everything was just as smooth as silk.

"Didn't you get the photos I sent you?" I asked him.

"No, I didn't have time to go through all my emails."

"Didn't anyone from the ER contact you about my infection? Plus, I've developed this awful ringing in my ears. It seems to get worse every time I use the device."

"No, no one told me there was any issue until Deni called."

I lifted up my shirt.

Dr. Dandico and the student he was training voiced an extremely loud, "Holy cow! Would you look at that!"

Ben Dales and B. B. Beaudreaux

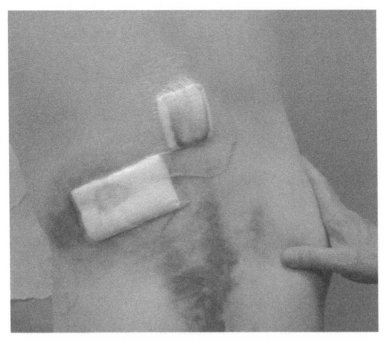

Taken post-implant by a medical student of Dr. Dandico.

"Oh, I've seen it." I said.

"Well, you should have told me it was like this," Dr. Dandico retorted.

"I sent you photos. I was very, very sick. I was so sick with acute respiratory infection that I thought I was going to die. Even the ER doctor thought so. Didn't anyone report this to you?"

"No, no, no one told me anything about this. But it just looks like we may have hit a blood vessel," he said. "This should clear up in a few weeks."

I raised my eyebrows. "You hit a blood vessel at both surgical sites?"

"Yes. It's not uncommon, and you can see it's clearing up already."

Looking back, this comment was so ironic. Dr. Dandico had not seen the photos to begin with, so how could he know it was clearing up already?

Admittedly, I was in too much of a stupor to argue the point at the time. Since he was part of a teaching hospital network, Dr. Dandico had his student take more photographs of the bruises. After the appointment, I asked the student to send me the photos. Had he not sent them at that very moment, those photos surely never would have made it to my email account.

Something was very seriously wrong, but it was dealt with as if I merely had a minor complication.

As I continued to see Dr. Dandico following the implant, I started hearing questions from the medical device company's representative whenever he would come to the appointments.

"Does the battery area ever feel warm?"

"Of course it does. I told my doctor about this from the start. Every time I charge the device, it gets hot."

Ben Dales and B. B. Beaudreaux

"Well, how are you charging it?"

"When I am lying down in bed."

"Why don't you charge it while lying on your side, so that air can get to it?" He suggested.

I also explained that the device would never stay fully charged even if I charged it and did not turn it on. My biggest complaint, however, after the bruising and then the infection that sent me to the emergency room, was the tinnitus I was suffering. At first, the tinnitus appeared shortly after I turned on the device, but the more I used it, the more prevalent the tinnitus became.

At every appointment, Dr. Dandico kept telling me there was nothing wrong. But I knew it was heating up, and the tinnitus was becoming unbearable. Two years later, I finally hit my limit with the lack of answers.

"It's idiopathic," Dr. Dandico told me, meaning they didn't know why the tinnitus was happening.

"No, it's not," I insisted. "I never had tinnitus before. It's because of this device. Get this thing out of me. Get it out, I don't care. I don't care what the reps are telling you, that there's nothing wrong, that 'it'll get better,' no. It's just getting worse. It never did what it was supposed to do."

Dr. Dandico finally scheduled the device explant after I told him to get it out of me. We had gone through two years of appointments in which I insisted something was wrong, only to be told nothing was wrong.

Looking back, I now know that there were behind-the-scenes safety concerns about the mini-neurostimulator nearly from the onset, because this newer and more compact device employed a smaller battery. The reason the battery pack was "so much smaller" and was consequently being deemed as an "easy procedure" was simple: the company had changed from a regular battery to the new lithium-ion battery.

Had my doctor and the device company's representative not questioned me, it would have taken me more time to figure out that the battery in the device was burning me from within the entire time it was inside me.

Ben Dales and B. B. Beaudreaux

CHAPTER 25

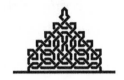

Deni: The Tinnitus Test

Ted had to undergo a trial run of having the neurostimulator battery device implanted in his back. He had to have a couple of lead wires inserted into his back connected to an external battery pack that he wore on his belt. This was not to be a hospital procedure but rather done during an office visit with his primary pain doctor. This was intended to give him a chance to see how the permanent mini-neurostimulator would be able to help him alleviate the constant pain which he was enduring.

The results had been somewhat inconclusive. His main reaction to this pre-implant procedure had been that the leads inserted into his back with the rods that shocked his dura had given him a new constant painful irritation, causing him to up his dosage of medication for this "test" surgery. He likened it to shoving a thermometer into a piece of meat to see if it was finished cooking. Therefore, it may have diverted him from thinking so much about his chronic leg pains to thinking about the new pain in his back from these leads.

The day of the implant, I arranged to arrive at school late in order to drive Ted to the hospital. This was to be a bit more serious a procedure than the earlier one when the test battery pack was put into his back. He forewarned me it would consequently be a full day at the hospital for him. Dr. Dandico would need three or more hours to accomplish the implant, to be followed by a few hours of recuperation time for Ted at the hospital. However, we were told that most likely he would not be admitted for an overnight stay.

I finished out my teaching day and dashed to my car immediately after clocking out from school. I recall making good time to the northside hospital, since I was driving a tad before the start of rush hour. When I arrived, Ted was still slightly in a groggy state in the recovery area but was being released to go home right away. This was a good thing, as rush hour was still in its beginning stages, and we were able to make it home without the heavy delays there would be later.

After dropping him off in order that he could

Ben Dales and B. B. Beaudreaux

go straight to bed, I scurried on to our local pharmacy to drop off his prescriptions. This gave me a chance to swing by a favorite local restaurant to get a couple of "comfort food" dinners to bring home. After picking up his filled prescriptions, I headed home with the hot food so that he could partake of both before resting for the evening.

His pain level was not horrible at the time, although admittedly he was filled with ample medications. He was lucid enough, though, to be able to try out charging his newly-implanted neurostimulator. It was largely a non-event, although I do recall his sharing that it seemed to be very warm internally for him.

The next day and each subsequent day, I returned home from school curious of his condition. My hopes for his daily recovery showing improvement were not being fulfilled, but instead he was feeling worse each day. This was something for which we were not prepared. It got to the point that he was feeling so badly, we decided we could not even chance driving way up to the northside to see his doctor. We had to go to the ER of the closest hospital to our home. This turned out to be harrowing in itself, even more than one expects from a typical ER visit. He was diagnosed with a severe respiratory infection. This, combined with the widespread bluish-purple bruising in his back made the ER quite frankly wonder if he was dying. One staff member asked us if Ted would want to be admitted or would simply like to undergo his future at home. Fearful upon hearing this reaction, we still opted for the latter.

Back home, we contacted Dr. Dandico's office the next day with emailed photos and a telephone message as follow-up. An appointment was made for the following week, as we had been advised to fill some new prescriptions for the respiratory infection and give them a chance to work.

By the time Ted went to see Dr. Dandico for his appointment, the infection problem was reduced. The bruising in his back, however, was most definitely not.

Although it was good that finally Dr. Dandico got to see and hear firsthand what Ted was going through, it did not really seem to sink in how awfully the prior week had gone.

During the weeks and months that followed, there were more follow-up appointments with Dr. Dandico and with a SAN representative. Although the problems identified during the ER visit seemed to lessen, there were still ongoing concerns-- primarily the heat being generated inside his body whenever the device was being charged and continuing afterwards. Another concern was

Ben Dales and B. B. Beaudreaux

something new, that of ringing in the ears. These were reported and monitored during subsequent doctor visits, the latter of which was identified as tinnitus.

I was able to participate in some of these doctor visits and came away with a few observations. Those involving Dr. Dandico, I largely recall his trying to be interested in hearing Ted's concerns and in being positive about each prognosis for the future. Those involving SAN representatives were more troubling. The first representative was a man, Galli Vincente, who seemed competent and genuine in hearing what Ted had to say. He always asked a lot of questions, especially about the heat being generated by his company's device implanted in Ted's back. The most troubling part, however, was that after a year of these meetings with him, he disappeared.

Without any advance notice, we were told at an appointment by Dr. Dandico and by a new SAN representative that he had left the company--that was it, no other explanation. Not only disappointed, we were somewhat devastated by this news. Here was someone we had come to trust and confide in who exited our lives without warning. The new representative was a young woman who, as we quickly learned, was quite inexperienced. During that very first meeting, it was Ted who had to show her how to use the charger and explain the process of how it worked.

As for the permanent mini-neurostimulator, Ted had wanted the thing out of him since shortly after it had been implanted. There had been repercussions with it that never went away but instead just seemed to worsen. The most noticeable perhaps, and certainly the one he had complained about the most, was the ringing in his ears--tinnitus. A secondary one had been the heat generated from within his body around the device, although as it turned out, this should be termed the primary one. It was the one that broke the proverbial camel's back.

The horrible, constant ringing in his ears seemed to be more pronounced in the city, almost as if exacerbated by cell phone usage. Ted told me was usually at a pitch of A flat. However, he also shared that there were times when he could hear ringing related to people's phones somewhere out in the proverbial cloud. He and eventually I came to believe that the city's widespread and constant communications signals were directly affecting his tinnitus and the wide range of signals his hearing seemed to be intercepting while the device was inside his body.

Eventually we decided to put this theory to a little test. We began taking small road trips out

Ben Dales and B. B. Beaudreaux

of the city. As we did so, it seemed to him that the extraneous signals were lessened. Finally, we decided to try another test. Our plan was to spend some periods of time staying at Ted's grandparents' country house up in the northwoods of Wisconsin. This place was so remote that our cell phones could only get a signal by our going to the upstairs bedroom and holding the phone out the window. Getting any sort of computer connection was impossible. Heck, the house still had a functioning dial phone, which not too many years prior was still part of a party line. We were eleven miles away from the nearest town. This being the largest town in the area, it had a population of some 1600 residents.

So yes, we were quite remote and quite free from all the radio and communication signals one experiences in the city.

Our test results were conclusive. His tinnitus and his reception of communication signals were greatly lessened. This caused us to start brainstorming ways we could get him out of the city on a more permanent basis. The two of us could not just pick up and move, due to my employment with the Chicago Public Schools. The city mandates that all city employees, including teachers, must live within the confines of the city. All we could do was get away when school was not in session, such as summers and breaks. We did seriously consider moving Ted farther somewhere out of the city during the school year, yet still close enough that I would be able to get away each weekend to be with him. This never really panned out for us, which is another major reason that he (and we) eventually opted for the removal of the device from his body.

The long-awaited explant surgery was scheduled at last. With the removal already on our calendar, the mini-neurostimulator recall letter appeared in our mailbox.

Ben Dales and B. B. Beaudreaux

CHAPTER 26

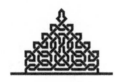

Ted: The Recall

I realize now that the explant surgery was a sweep-it-under-the-rug moment more than anything. If I had any doubt about the removal of the neurostimulator, it vanished as soon as I opened the recall letter in the mail.

Dear Patient: St. Jude Medical is providing patients and physicians with important information about their Eon and Eon Mini Charging Systems (Models: 3701, 3711, and 3721).

In a letter dated December 19, 2011, St. Jude Medical informed physicians of patient complaints of warmth or heating at the implant site during charging for the Eon and Eon Mini spinal cord stimulators. Your physician may have informed you of the letter and the recommendations to avoid uncomfortable heating. This letter provides you with our current and expanded recommendations on how to reduce heating while charging the spinal cord stimulator and an update of patient complaints. We are also providing the same recommendations to your physician.

As you know, the Charging System is used to charge your spinal cord stimulator for the management of your chronic pain. St. Jude Medical has informed your doctor that a number of cases have been reported in which discomfort associated with heating occurred at the device site while patients were using the Charging System to charge their spinal cord stimulator. In three cases, patients received a burn to the skin (one second-degree and two first-degree burns) at the implant site. This information applies only to the specific model of the charging systems listed above. Our records indicate that you may have one of these charging systems. During charging, it is normal to feel an increase in temperature at the implant site; however, you should not feel pain or discomfort. In most cases, patients do not report an uncomfortable temperature increase during charging; however, some patients have reported uncomfortable or intolerable temperature elevations. St. Jude Medical has received 325 total patient complaints of warmth or heating at the device implant site during charging for the Eon and Eon Mini spinal cord stimulation systems, which equates to 0.46% of total implants as of June 30, 2012. Some physicians or patients have

Ben Dales and B. B. Beaudreaux

requested explant surgery to address uncomfortable temperature elevations. These reports resulted in a total of 72 explants for the Eon and Eon Mini spinal cord stimulators, or a rate of 0.10% of total implants. Explant surgery, as with any surgery, presents a risk to health. Adverse events associated with an unplanned surgery may be comparable to adverse events associated with planned operations and may include pain, scarring, and infection as well as complications from anesthesia.

The second page of the recall was filled with battery charging recommendations and wrapped up with: "We regret any concerns this may cause you and your family."

The recall letter simply validated what I had suspected for awhile--the unit was not functioning properly. I wanted to keep the neurotransmitter once it was removed. I wanted to know what was really going on.

I was not surprised it was being recalled. It felt strange, though, that the device was being recalled right out of my own body (as it was from countless others). Only then did everything fall a bit more quickly into place.

I felt like I had been duped. The more I later learned about the bigger picture, the more this feeling became fact.

With the ongoing advice of the SAN representative, my doctor agreed to allow the device that was burning me from within to stay in my body for more than a year while the damage was being done.

CHAPTER 27

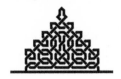

Ted: The Confrontation

When I arrived at the hospital that morning, I wrote on the hospital release form my own specific instructions for the hospital and its staff, including Dr. Dandico. My handwritten and signed instructions were that the neurostimulator was to be given to me after surgery. My reasoning was that the device had been purchased for me by my insurance when I consented to have it implanted. It had been part of my body and rightfully belonged to me. Therefore I wanted it. The reason for this is simple: it was the key to my proving that the unit had been malfunctioning.

After I was already on the gurney and feeling the early effects of the sedation, Dr. Dandico came to speak with me. I had in my hand a copy of the release with my handwritten and signed modification stating the actual device was to be saved and given back to me. I told him to make sure the unit was not discarded with other medical waste.

"Oh, the device company's people are in the operating room waiting for you," he said.

Hearing this, I was both shocked and incensed. "What are they doing in there?"

"They want to see the explant surgery."

Being under sedation, I had to take a moment to think about the other parts of the release that I signed. It did say that the hospital was a teaching facility, where medical students sometimes are in the gallery. But...that did not mean I had agreed to allow corporate non-physician people gawking at me while they cut me open.

I had shown Dr. Dandico a copy of the release, which I had his receptionist copy just for him so that he would know these were my instructions and to provide proof they were on file with the hospital. I told him to make sure I got that device, because I wanted to have independent testing done on it to prove what I had been claiming about it the entire time.

"I don't know if I can do that."

"What do you mean? It's my device," I blurted out as the sedation was taking even more effect.

Ben Dales and B. B. Beaudreaux

However, as we were still discussing that (and debating what would become of my device), one of the medical students who went by the name of Ahmed came over to talk to Dr. Dandico and me. In so doing, he had forgotten to take off his mask that had been pulled down around his throat when he left the previous surgery.

Dr. Dandico literally flipped out. He turned his attention to Ahmed's oversight.

"Is that your mask from the previous surgery?"

Ahmed then realized with a sheepish expression that it was, just as Dandico started screaming at him, "What the fuck are you doing, trying to spread germs through the entire fucking hospital?! Take that fucking thing off right now and don't ever, ever come out of one surgery to the other with the same garments on!"

I had never heard Dr. Dandico blow his top before, so it was unexpected. Nevertheless, I turned back to my concerns, and I reiterated that it was my device--the one that I bought, the one that is supposed to go home with me.

"I don't want the representatives in the room."

As I was staring fervently at him, Dr. Dandico was not looking me in the eye.

"Start it." He told the anesthesiologist.

Looking back now, I believe there was more to Dr. Dandico's surprisingly loud, profane, and furious outburst than just anger at this medical student. I was full of questions.

Was Dr. Dandico not only being manipulated but also blackmailed due to some nondisclosure agreements he may have signed earlier with the company?

Were the representatives of that very company in the OR just "to watch," or really to make sure that the device went nowhere but back to the company that made it?

Was the neurostimulator device company forcing Dr. Dandico to do things its way?

Once again, I felt like bolting out of that operating room, but there were two reasons I could not. The first was that I was already going under, due to the IV drip in my arm. The second was that the device **had to be taken out of me.** Since I was already sedated and on the gurney, what else could I do about it at the time? I felt like I had just been run over by a steamroller and that everyone in that operating room was part of the coordinated conspiracy to keep the truth from me, including the physician I had literally trusted

Ben Dales and B. B. Beaudreaux

with my life for nearly a decade. How could he live with himself? As I was going under, all I could think about was what he would have done had this neurostimulator been installed in one of his own children. We had such a personal relationship that I actually knew the name of his wife and children. I felt betrayed.

Of course the "company people" were in the operating room for one reason: to abscond with the device. There was indeed nothing I was able to do about it.

No one from that company talked to me afterwards. It was a complete boondoggle. The company took my device because they knew they were going to be sued, and my doctor, with whom I trusted my life, let them walk away with it. This is when I realized that Dr. Dandico was complying with, or at the very least, was being coerced by this company.

The entire surgery took quite a bit longer than anticipated. When Dr. Dandico made the first incision, he made a shocking discovery: the neurostimulator device itself was encased within my back in a hard rubbery scar tissue substance.

For two long years, the lithium-ion battery was burning inside of me.

Dr. Dandico now faced a very complicated process to remove the neurostimulator. He had to cut the metal rods out of me, literally by slicing through the hard rubbery scar tissue encasing them. To remove the battery pack, Dr. Dandico had to use force, meaning he literally had to use his own physical strength to force out the battery pack from the hard, rubbery scar tissue.

Once he removed the battery pack, Dr. Dandico still had the wire leads to extract from my body, since these leads were still connected to both the battery pack and the rods. Instead of cutting them out, he used pliers and started yanking on the wires from both ends until they were finally able to be extracted.

As it turned out, it took almost two extra hours in the surgery room. When Dr. Dandico verbalized his post-surgery summary to Deni, he was still perspiring from having to exert the strength he did to extract the neurostimulator components by force. However, I don't believe that was the only reason he was perspiring. I think he was nervous, and he used force that should not have been used on a human body to remove those components, especially the wires.

Additionally, Dr. Dandico could not avoid cutting through the scar tissue, having had to

Ben Dales and B. B. Beaudreaux

slice into me to cut out the rods connected to the neurostimulator from end to end. He had been unable to remove them via a simple small incision, such as was made when they were first implanted.

The end result on my body of the traumatic explant is captured in photos shared in this chapter.

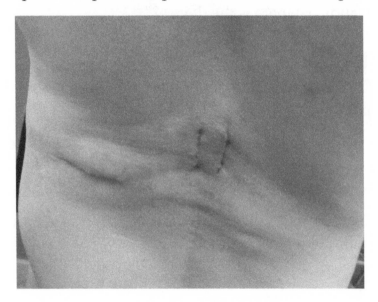

When I handed the doctor a copy of my request to keep the device, I had another copy tucked inside my wallet in the locker that had been provided for me to put my clothes and valuables in as I changed into a surgical gown. I still have that copy, and have since scanned it online and uploaded it into the cloud for others to view.

I do have some parting comments about the actions of the SAN Medical Device Company representatives not only being allowed by Dr. Dandico in the room during my surgery, but also about how he allowed them to take the neurostimulator device, which was rightfully mine.

The first thing I asked when I came to was, "Dr. Dandico, where is the device?"

"Well, I think it was taken up to pathology."

"Pathology? It's not human tissue, what would pathology do with it?"

"Others need to look at it."

"You mean SAN Medical has it."

"They're obligated to test it to see if it was malfunctioning."

"I'm supposed to believe them?"

It was at that exact moment I completely lost faith in him as a physician who was truly looking out for me. He was the top person in charge. He could have made sure that that device went from the OR to me. There was no pathology to be done on it since it was not living tissue. Even if there was pathology to be done on it, then it should have gone to the pathology lab and not to the hands of the representatives. My trust in him was broken, because I figured he knew that I knew he had been pulled into causing severe trauma--all in the name of profits for the medical device company. My faith in the entire human race changed that very moment and to this day, I have a hard time trusting people.

CHAPTER 28

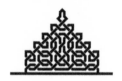

Deni: The Removal

U nlike the day of the implant surgery nearly two years ago, I decided to accompany Ted to the hospital and to wait for him to finish the whole ordeal. His surgeon had predicted that it might take up to two hours for the explant to be accomplished and for him to be in a state to return home. It was going to require him to "go under completely," so additional time might be required for him to "come out of it" and be able to travel.

I was with him in the pre-surgery area, where different individuals reviewed what exactly was going to happen with him and then requested his signature on the various consent forms. Although this part may often be a cut-and-dried, relatively short process with many individuals, this was never the case with Ted. He had always read and reviewed all the details of these standard forms, and he usually makes changes as he deems

Ben Dales and B. B. Beaudreaux

necessary before signing anything. In fact, he had taught me always to do the same (which I have done ever since). It is significant to note here that on one of the forms, he amended it to read that since the device became his property at the time of the implant that he was ordering it to be returned to him after surgery for his own independent study and research of it.

Ted was ushered away to the surgery room while I was instructed where the waiting room was (which as it turned out, seemed to be in a different part of the hospital...or at least suffice it to say, it was not nearby). There was coffee available there, and I had brought my own snacks and a book to read. I settled in for a couple of hours to wait, during which I observed and learned the routine of the waiting room from the matron in charge.

As it turned out, my own wait got to the point that it was exceeding not only the two hours predicted, but reached three hours. I was not yet panicking but I decided to excuse myself for a bit (and I told the matron the same), and proceeded to walk back without permission to the surgery area. Herein I learned that Ted was still in surgery. I quietly returned to the waiting room area.

Finally, after more than four hours of waiting, Dr. Dandico came to the desk to ask for me. We had gotten to know each other during Ted's many previous appointments. He approached me and smiled, even if it seemed to me a bit forced. I was nervous, to say the least.

His first words were, "Ted is all right and is just being taken into recovery. The explant was a success."

He then told me he wished to tell me all about it and suggested we go to one of the smaller consultation rooms adjacent to the waiting area. I agreed, though I was feeling a bit apprehensive about what I was going to hear.

After we entered the room, he closed the door and suggested that we both sit. I took out my notebook and pen and advised that I needed to take notes to use where and when my memory might fail me. He smiled and concurred it would be a good idea.

"Everything is all right," he immediately began, "Ted is doing fine."

I watched as his face became a bit more concerned and serious. He told me that there had been some difficulties in the removal of the device itself. He admitted how surprised, if not shocked, he was once he opened Ted up to remove the neurostimulator. He stated he had expected the usual amount of scar tissue surrounding the

Ben Dales and B. B. Beaudreaux

device but instead found the device encased in an extremely hard and unexpectedly rubber-like scar tissue. He told me he was forced to slice through this hard rubbery tissue, which of course complicated the surgery even more.

As it was, Dr. Dandico said he did in fact have to spend an extra two hours just struggling to remove by force the wires to the rods that ran from the battery pack of the neurostimulator. He shared that it was a slow, tedious, and damaging process. The damage, he stated, was in the fact that the neurostimulator had internally burned the surrounding tissue to the point that it had literally hardened into a hard rubbery substance. This produced massive hemorrhaging at the implant sites.

In hindsight, that was what was causing the bruising and the infection of the tissue surrounding the battery pack and the two electrodes in the thoracic area of the dura. He further shared he was grateful that he did not have to resort to slicing through this substance more than was needed for removal of the wire leads attached to the device. He continued to share the extreme difficulties he faced in removing the device by sheer force, stating he was almost physically unable to do so.

As a result, he told me that he was extremely concerned about Ted's physical condition after going through this internal trauma. In fact, right on the spot, Dr. Dandico mandated that I agree to be very vigilant of Ted's post-surgery condition and that I would not hesitate to drive him to the nearest emergency room in case of any signs whatsoever of complications.

"Do you have any questions?"

"Yes, I do," I replied. "When will we have to come back to have his stitches removed?"

Dr. Dandico paused for a second or two. "I know this is going to sound hard to believe, because I cannot even believe it myself, but there was no need for stitches or staples."

"But how could that be?" I asked in shock.

He looked me straight in the eyes. "The areas where the components were in his body were so encased in scar tissue that, even though I had to dig those pieces out, nothing bled."

"That's absurd, Doctor!" I couldn't hold back. "How can you have removed that device and just told me all the problems you had trying to remove it, and not need to sew the exact same area where you used staples when you implanted the device?"

With a resigned look, he began to explain.

"There was so much rubbery tissue surrounding not just the battery pack, but all around the rods that were placed right against his dura, that even the large incisions I had to make to excise the device didn't cause any bleeding. Somehow the scar tissue just kept building up and building up around this entire surgical site. I've never seen anything like it before," he admitted. "I'm thinking I'm going to have to write a paper on this anomaly."

"Did the device cause this?"

"It must have," he responded. "There is no other way for me to account for what happened here."

"Is it bandaged?"

"There is some overlay on it. He won't have to return to have any stitches removed, because there aren't any, as I said. Just keep an eye on it."

"I will."

CHAPTER 29

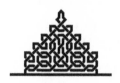

Ted: Researching Even Deeper

The latest and greatest phone that everyone was talking about at the time was a steal-- literally. One mega company (legally) stole it from another mega company. This was clear from the very beginning of its introduction. The physical similarities were the same. The Operating System of this latest phone, although different from the one it copied, still had the same functionality. One other startling similarity was the type of batteries it was using.

Lithium-ion batteries were known to pack a huge amount of power into a small amount of space. These batteries were smaller and lighter with more power to go longer distances and longer times without being recharged. The problem, though, was that of a decrease in the safety component from the onset. It has now become common knowledge that when lithium-ion batteries are charged and

Ben Dales and B. B. Beaudreaux

recharged, they can generate enough heat to cause explosions. Widely publicized, this has been the case with hoverboards, e-cigarettes and lighters, various cell phones, and electric cars. A United Parcel Service plane crashed when a cargo of lithium-ion batteries caught fire, killing the crew. In any case, all of these types of devices carried a high amount of risk for fires.

If you research the link between fires and lithium-ion batteries that surfaced during 2015, you can find a vast amount of content on this very subject from many consumers. Although this revelation has since become drastically clear with the introduction of the Samsung Galaxy phone, it was not so clear back in the time of the newly-marketed neurostimulators (around 2010). This was simply due to supply and demand. The public demand was not that high for neurostimulator devices, even though profits were through the roof. Many insurance carriers did not cover the cost of the device and the surgery that went with it.

One report helping me see the bigger picture about SAN Medical was in the August 2, 2012 issue of Becker's Healthcare publication called Becker's ASC Review. Its "Pain Management" section in that issue revealed that this company "...is recalling some of its...pain management implants due to battery and charging issues, according to a Mass

Device report...The company received reports that the batteries in the neurostimulation devices failed early or overheated during recharging, at times leaving patients with first- or second-degree burns."

Now one has to wonder why it took so long for this news to be made public--some two years after my recall letter had been mailed to me.

Since then, it has become public information about other recalls of medical devices due to these same types of batteries. In the publication *Drug Device*, Tabitha Kruger wrote an article for its October 13, 2016 issue that reported that the medical device maker "...has recalled some implantable defibrillators after a battery problem resulted in two patient deaths."

Further reports validated this. The *New York Post* edition dated April 13, 2017 included an article about the company that acquired the neurostimulator company in January of that year. The headline on this article read that this acquisition company "...must be getting a bad case of heartburn..." from its latest acquisition. The article stated that the "...medical device company got a warning letter from the Food and Drug Administration this week that detailed years of... failures to fix scary--and even deadly--defects in its implantable heart devices."

Ben Dales and B. B. Beaudreaux

It continued on to state that "Among the most egregious examples in the FDA's letter was this company's allowing seven patients to receive the company's implantable heart devices in late October--despite the company issuing a recall on the critical gadgets earlier that month due to a potentially fatal defect that could cause rapid battery depletion. To make matters worse, ten more of the faulty devices--whose defective batteries impaired their ability to deliver life-saving shock therapy--were sent to company field reps after the recall."

The battery change itself had been an easy one for the manufacturer with no clinical testing, because it was considered a "retrofit" part of a device that had already been approved.

No clinical testing. How is this even possible?

One large regulatory loophole is exposed in a 2018 article appearing in HealthNewsReview.org entitled, "Why 'approved' medical devices in the U.S. may not be safe or effective." Although the article offers much documentation and argument, one chapter sums it up. It states the following: Ninety-nine percent of devices never have to provide clinical data, thanks in part to the 2002 Medical Devices User Fee Act, which requires the FDA to use the "least burdensome route" to approval. That means most devices submit a 510(k), which has created a daisy chain of numerous modifications in which devices get tweaked and cleared for market without patient trials.

How did they pass the FDA requirements? How exactly do these medical device manufacturers do it?

Well, the pressuring influence of lobbyists is an obvious "guess." The multi-billion dollar medical device manufacturing industry pays its lobbyists to court those elected officials in Congress who are there to serve the people. These congresspeople, no matter their party, are then obligated to pass certain legislation at the hands of these lobbyists, pushed by the medical device industry. The impact then is not only limited to the private insurance network, but also impacts Medicare and Medicaid since our Congress oversees the FDA.

Apparently they do this with self-paid, self-peer reviews or with obvious lax oversight. This latter fact is what I have learned from various internet databases—including the *MAUDE database managed by the FDA—devoted to keeping track of malfunctioning medical devices, dangerous medications, unscrupulous or unethical physicians, surgeons, large medical groups, hospitals, and higher-level learning institutions.

Ben Dales and B. B. Beaudreaux

One such database quotes the *New York Times* editorial from May 4, 2019 ("80,000 Deaths. 2 Million Injuries. It's time for a Reckoning on Medical Devices."), that clarifies this very issue in its statement, "It seems incredible that products meant to reside inside the human body would be used on patients without any proof of safety or efficacy. But thanks to regulatory loopholes and lax oversight, most medical devices are poorly vetted before their release into the marketplace and poorly monitored after the fact."

The 2002 Medical Devices User Fee Act we mentioned allows for a daisy chain of numerous modifications in which medical devices get tweaked and cleared for market without patient trials. In other words, any modification to a previously-approved device can simply be cleared for use without any documentation attesting to its effectiveness, or more importantly, its safety to the patient.

This type of modification without approval or testing is what happened in my case with the neurostimulator. The original battery used in this device was replaced with the lithium-ion battery that burned me from within. It had neither been tested nor approved, yet was cleared to do its damage to me and, I would guess, countless others.

The same *NYT* editorial from May 4, 2019 also includes the reasons for delays in removing faulty medical devices from a person's body as well as from the entire market. The article states, "Problems can take years to emerge and can be impossible to correct, in part because permanent implants are not easily extracted from the body.... When trouble does arise, device makers often equivocate, regulators dither, and patients seeking redress are forced into lengthy and expensive court battles. In the end, faulty products can remain on the market for years."

Finally the article concludes with a haunting statement of the effects of waiting for faulty medical devices to be removed:

"The risks of waiting loom large: in the past decade, nearly two million injuries and more than 80,000 deaths have been linked to faulty medical devices, many approved with little to no clinical testing, according to a global investigation by the International Consortium of Investigative Journalists."

It is a frightening revelation that these companies are inadvertently testing their devices upon us, the unsuspecting members of the public, creating life-and-death situations--all for the purpose of making money.

Ben Dales and B. B. Beaudreaux

We are paying health insurance premiums plus the required copay amounts, along with whatever is not covered by insurance. Meanwhile, these insurance companies are approving the medical device implantations. Our physicians are telling them (and us) this is the best course of treatment, even though they do not have true facts or research statistics proving it is the best treatment. This is compounded even when components within the devices are literally switched to create often an entirely new device without any testing or oversight. In other words, the medical device manufacturers are literally twisting the arms of surgeons and physicians in an effort to keep products rolling out of the laboratories and into patients without the effectiveness ever being fully tested or known. Long-term effects are not understood. Devices that have been on the market for long periods of time can be redesigned without any testing and yet somehow make their way into the operating room, and into the patient.

This is exactly what happened to me when the company that provided the neurostimulator changed the type of battery to a lithium-ion battery. When minimal or no oversight is brought into any medical advancement (such as a new medical device), problems become more likely.

My story is a blatant example of this. Even if

there were peer reviews by other entities, how biased does one think they might be? These companies spent millions of dollars in research, and they certainly were not going to miss out on getting a financial return--at least a return on their initial investment to cover the costs associated with research and development. They also needed financial return to appease their stockholders in order that others would continue to invest in these very companies, no matter what happened in trials with animals.

This is simply another prime example of how health care has become the single biggest sector of the U.S. economy.

The important thing to note about animal trials is that animals cannot explain what is wrong. Animals might have reactions and they might survive the trials, but they cannot tell you what else may be going on. Only humans can share things such as, "This burns..." or "This makes my ears keep ringing nonstop..." or even, "This is bothering me in a different way now...." When it comes to issues, it is easy for workers in a lab to overlook a potential problem that has surfaced in a test animal, because if they do not get these devices into timely production, they will not have a job.

A sad sidelight to these animal test subjects is that once a result is concluded, these animals serve no further purpose whatsoever. They cannot be used again for other research, since they have become "tainted" due to their having been used previously on a different type of testing. Therefore, these animals are euthanized. Laboratories have no reason to keep previously-tested animals around for the rest of their lifetimes. Unless the testing is for a long-term study of a particular medication, research animals are deemed an expense.

It is obvious that the word "expense" carries the most negative connotation among those charged with the testing of any new medical device, procedure, or drug. The goal is simply to secure the revered and necessary FDA approval while spending the least amount of money to do so. The bottom line is critical among the many stockholders whose monies financially support the research.

A lesson never learned? Or is it that the correct lesson is still being overruled by the bottom line for the medical industry?

*MAUDE Database: https://www.accessdata. fda.gov/scripts/cdrh/cfdocs/cfMAUDE/search. CFM

CHAPTER 30

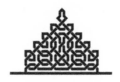

Ted: After Removal

After the malfunctioning neurostimulator was removed, things did not get any better. I still had tinnitus. The pain in both legs was never-ending. I also started suffering from what I could only describe as a swollen tongue. Initially I thought it was caused by the toothpaste I was using. There had been so many new formulas of toothpaste on the market claiming to be whitening this and enameling that, I decided to switch to baking soda to combat my swollen tongue. But the switch failed to solve the problem.

Once again I found myself contacting my general practitioner, Dr. Lottens, with whom I maintained a cordial relationship for several years. I sent him a photo of my tongue. He wrote back suggesting I come in for a checkup.

Ben Dales and B. B. Beaudreaux

In the meantime, I started researching on the internet what this might be. Here I learned it was a condition called "geographic tongue." There had not been much determination in the medical community about the causes of this condition-- just as there was not much on tinnitus causes. My doctor told me that these were all symptoms of an underlying problem and that they were poorly understood in the medical community. As I delved more into the reasons of these bizarre symptoms, it all came back to my previous diagnosis of Adhesive Arachnoiditis.

I had a huge learning curve to get to the point of understanding this disease. But as I read the book, I more readily understood what had happened to me during not only the first surgery using the bone growth stimulator, but also what happened during the surgery that was intended to correct the failed partial fusion that was initially attempted. Not only were my nerve roots stuck together, so was the entire cauda columna. The neurostimulator that burned me from the inside out merely knocked me from the frying pan into the fire.

Since Adhesive Arachnoiditis is a degenerative disease, things get progressively worse no matter how carefully anyone with this disease walks the line. There has to be a meticulous balance between taking the proper amount of medication to control the pain and getting enough physical therapy to keep the affected limbs from atrophying. The catch-22 is that the more one uses the muscles that are affected--in my case, my legs--the more they involuntarily fasciculate or undulate because the muscles themselves think they are getting signals from the brain to fire. So too much exercise will cause one's legs to cramp up, and they will atrophy anyway.

Most nights I just lie awake in bed with thoughts of all the things that went wrong. And always: Was there something I could have or should have done? But the fact is, it was all a set-up.

That's right, I was set up.

The surgeons who were "courted" by the medical electronic device manufacturers were lied to by these very manufacturers. These manufacturing corporations needed to recoup their development costs. There is a separation, if not a huge divide, between the representatives of the corporation and the patient. A patient's welfare is not their primary concern. A patient represents dollar signs to them. The bottom line is their primary concern.

When a company's research and development people create a product, the corporation will do anything to have its costs reimbursed. Otherwise,

Ben Dales and B. B. Beaudreaux

if there is no use for the product, all that money is wasted. So even when the reviews are inconclusive, the corporation does not care. Quite frankly, that is why the medical corporations have paid a select group of physicians to submit positive peer reviews. If physicians want to keep getting paid by these corporations, they have to keep telling the corporations that the devices are effective--even when they are not.

That last statement is not an opinion. Far too many patients have been subjected to failed medical devices and the documentation exists.

What is far too many?

An editorial in the May 4, 2019, edition of the *New York Times* that we previously mentioned reveals some startling numbers. The headline of the story reads, "80,000 Deaths. 2 Million Injuries. It's Time for a Reckoning on Medical Devices." The story's byline continues with "Patients suffer as the F.D.A. fails to adequately screen or monitor products."

Much of what so many of us have been told about the medical system in the U.S. is complete fallacy. Some of the "paid-for-hire" physicians do not care an iota about the health of patients. They have been trained to behave in this manner because all physicians will have patients who will eventually die. They are taught to be able to disassociate themselves from the death or suffering of a patient. The system is geared for them simply to move on to the next patient.

After all, there is more money to be made, and very little money is apt to be made on a patient who is going to die soon anyway.

The reason they are taught to act this way in medical school is because these medical schools are being funded by pharmaceutical companies, by insurance companies, and yes--by the medical electronic device manufacturers. It would be great to think that medical schools are teaching their students to make sure that there is nothing more important than the patient. But since tuition alone would barely cover the cost of professor salaries, the medical schools around the world look to third-party benefactors to subsidize their needed funding. This of course is a dangerous game, because obviously the corporations that fund them are only looking to make more money for their investors.

But the truth is, insurance companies do not primarily exist to save us from crippling lives or horrible diseases or untimely deaths. Insurance companies exist because they are making a bet that most people will pay insurance premiums their entire lives without a sniffle until around age

Ben Dales and B. B. Beaudreaux

65, when they get run over by a bus or something similarly fatal happens. There is little regard for the welfare of the general public. Corporate executives make big money by not paying claims. There are even bonuses for the executives who keep costs down to a minimum.

This in turn means that the person who needs a bone marrow transplant because they have lymphoma will not be approved for the procedure. This is not because it will not cure them, but because it would be a huge expense for the insurance company. These companies will insist that bone marrow transplants are "experiments" and do not fall under the standard means of treatment protocol. Of course this is a lie, and there are some doctors who know this and even a few who will admit it. The only problem is that most doctors are controlled by these corporations because they know that the less money the insurance companies pay out, the more money they will take home in bonuses.

A physician friend of mine once shared confidentially with me how treatment of patients is allocated. The insurance companies advise physicians there is an allotted pool of insurance money per physician. If all allotted money is used, then that's it and there is no more. If less than the allotted money is used, all physicians in that particular physicians' group will receive bonuses. Finally, if more money is used than is allowed than is allowed in the pool, then less money will be available the next year for patients who use their services, even if it is warranted.

As far as "good" insurance goes, this is also a mixed bag. I long thought that having the "best" insurance was of the utmost importance. As it has turned out for me, having the best has qualified me to have more invasive procedures, which can be billed at higher rates than people who have less expensive insurance. This is another type of catch-22. If I hadn't had insurance that would pay for the bone growth stimulator to be used, my surgical physician would have had to use my own bone as seed material for the original fusion. This was the tried-and-true method that had been used so many times previously and had worked.

But my insurance would pay more, simply if the diagnostic code matched the corresponding procedure code. This had been pre-approved by my insurance company, so that a larger amount could be billed by the physicians' group. That is exactly why they used this procedure on me.

Ben Dales and B. B. Beaudreaux

CHAPTER 31

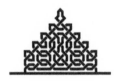

Deni: After Removal

With Ted back home ready for eventual recuperation, we nestled in to do everything possible to make it happen. We knew it was not all going to happen overnight. Our primary goal was to relieve him of leftover pain from the explant surgery.

The first step--rest and nutrition. I had secured his prescribed post-op medications from our neighborhood pharmacy, so we immediately began that routine in combination with food as advised. I tried to keep him in bed or at rest as much as possible and brought his meals to him. His follow-up appointment with his explant surgeon was in ten days, so we were hoping and praying there would be some signs of improvement by that time.

There was not. His tinnitus continued. The post-op pain was not leaving his body as hoped.

We went to his appointment together some ten days later to meet with Dr. Dandico. We of course reported the lack of progress toward recuperation. He listened intently and then asked for our patience, telling us that recovery and recuperation time is different from patient to patient. He requested that we stay in touch but to come see him again in a month.

We did see him again in a month and then on a consistent monthly basis afterwards. Of course, the monthly appointments were required in order to be able to have his needed prescriptions updated and filled each month.

As time went on and we were asked once again by the doctor to be patient during the recuperation and hopefully the improvement period, we gradually came to realize the damages done by the implant and subsequent explant of the neurostimulator were not going away. The existence of the lasting damages was extremely disappointing, particularly the resulting tinnitus that continued as if the device were still a part of his body, but it also helped us toward another major decision.

Ben Dales and B. B. Beaudreaux

We needed to move to the country, something which finally was going to be possible for me for the first time in years. I was able to retire from teaching after the completion of the school year, and free at last to leave the city.

Although it would not be our ultimate retirement destination, we decided to make the old three-room farmhouse in the northwoods our first destination enroute to this dream. For the first time in years, there would be winter inhabitants in this small, creaky old house in the proverbial middle of nowhere.

The tinnitus was going to be put to its ultimate survival test.

There was one other glitch to solve. We would no longer be near his doctor and the nearby pharmacies that could respectively prescribe and dispense his required pain medications. We were at the mercy of the small town northwoods doctor who had served his grandparents when he was a kid and at times had even served his needs way back then.

Before making the move, we needed to visit this doctor, Dr. Holcomb Everett, after so many years to request his help. Ted collected all his files and photos of his condition, along with all the individual specifics of what went wrong during each time under the knife. When we went in to visit Dr. Everett's office for this really important (to us) consultation, we brought all the relevant "evidence" we could in order to show him. As it turned out, the old family doctor remembered Ted and his grandparents quite well and was more than willing to take over administering the prescriptions while we were in the northwoods.

This was the final step we needed to overcome in order to be at long last out of the city.

Ben Dales and B. B. Beaudreaux

CHAPTER 32

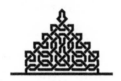

Ted: Lawsuits and More

After the fiasco with the mini-neurostimulator, I really started to think about all that happened to me.

I kept going back to the first surgery, when Dr. Clack performed a fusion with the help of a bone-growth stimulator device. I kept thinking about how I did not fuse on one side of the spinal processes. Now after all this time, the device itself was no longer on the market. I have since come to the conclusion that the bone growth stimulator was pulled from the market and immediately swept under the rug like so many other medical products that caused injury instead of doing what the manufacturers or producers claimed these products would.

What I do know from my studies of bone growth stimulators is that this type of electrical stimulation, for any type of wound or fusion, pulls the healing to one side--while at the same time, pulling it away from the other. One such study about electrical currents in the body, as documented in "The Electric Touch" article of the November 2017 issue of Discover, found that "The more that new tissue drew toward the current on one side of the wound, the more the other side recoiled."

The more I reflected on the first surgery and all the hidden information coming to light so many years later, the more I realized how much corruption is involved in the medical industry. I began to realize just how much control the medical device company had over my doctors. How much did Dr. Dandico really know about the medical device and the company that, if shared, could have prevented all the failures of the neurostimulator implant? Or Dr. Clack, for that matter? How many mistakes made, minute and monumental alike, are merely covered up and never discovered?

I decided to sue.

The law firm that originally represented me from the beginning of the lawsuit against the second medical device manufacturing company had sent my case on to another firm, which in turn, sent it out to still another law firm. I started getting calls, not from the attorneys I originally hired, but from

Ben Dales and B. B. Beaudreaux

other law firms I didn't even know. The attorneys had it in their contract--in some legal verbiage--that they could "farm out" my suit to other firms. It was not clear to me at the time and I came to realize that the attorneys I originally consulted did not have my best interest in mind.

No one from any of these firms thoroughly investigated what actually transpired in my particular case. No one inquired about the extent of the resulting injuries that happened specifically to me. Had they contacted me to research my case in detail, I could have explained and demonstrated in full. Of course they made it clear they had no such time or need to devote to this. Their representatives simply stated rather arrogantly and confidently that any further information I could offer would be unnecessary and was not going to be used.

The settlement amount was a pittance. Of course these attorneys headlined the offer amount as a whopping $32,000 and only added as a mere footnote that what the company was really offering me was this amount minus 40% for attorney fees plus all hidden costs, hidden expenses, and other undefined fees. This would have likely netted me a settlement of less than $12,000. I was shocked that the law firm I retained ended up offering such a small settlement amount.

$12,000...for a life totally ruined.

Moreover, in order to obtain the money, I was required to sign a non-disclosure agreement that in itself would have imposed upon me a gag order for the rest of my life or face being sued by the device manufacturer. How ironic. The medical manufacturers who caused this horrible tragic medical dilemma would be able to sue me. If I told anyone what this company's product did to me, I would be held legally responsible. Again, how ironic! The settlement amount was next to nothing for buying this kind of silence. Truly, the silence would be deafening.

With my resulting disability, I was no longer able to do much of anything anyway. What would have been the sense of accepting the pittance amount? Furthermore, since the initial disability was caused by the malfunctioning bone growth stimulator, that made it doubly so. No one would talk to me about the failure of that surgery either. When I started probing about the neurostimulator product, I similarly was told with little subtlety not to communicate with the doctors about what had happened to me.

Researching backward a bit, I was able to discover that there were ties between and among the group of attorneys that I had once consulted for myself in previous years, the device manufacturer, and this third party law firm (the one to which my

Ben Dales and B. B. Beaudreaux

case had been farmed out) that was now trying to get me to settle for that paltry amount. Although the money trail was almost impossible to follow, the idea that all these attorneys and this giant corporation were all corresponding together led me to the conclusion that this was yet another attempt to sweep it under the proverbial rug.

It was simply more profitable for everyone involved--that is, except for the injured person (me). Consequently I contacted two of the partners of the law firm where I had previously worked and with whom I was still in good standing when I left that firm. They told me that this particular company was a major client of theirs, and there was no way to assist me due to the alleged conflict of interest.

Of course I understood their predicament; they were worried they could be sued for conflict of interest at the very least. And they would have been! This device manufacturer had grown into a hundred-billion-dollar company, with long fingers reaching into everyone's pockets.

The contacts of attorneys with other attorneys are often vague on purpose. Automation has found ways of coding the exchange of information, of fees, and of client information and thus has virtually encrypted this information from anyone trying to learn about the covert communication and illegal activities between attorney partnerships and their respective clients. The only way to prove interaction between entities like these who are working together to sponsor corruption of the facts and dispel negativity about their products would have to be from an insider from either the law firm or from their pool of clients.

Finally, there are various people types out there, and just as money controlled an entire network of attorneys, there are enough intermediaries that would be willing to blow the whistle in order to recoup fraudulent spending by Medicare if they were not in fear of losing their jobs or getting into trouble themselves.

This opens up another whole can of worms. There are known lobbyists everywhere who are pushing these medical device products, pointing out supposed effectiveness based on self-peer reviews. In other words, these products are literally being pushed upon unsuspecting client patients just because of the unrelenting powerful forces such as lobbyists who are behind products that have little business being out there because they have very little proven effectiveness that can be trusted.

I have filed lawsuits against some of the physicians, and against SAN Medical Device Company, but I have not obtained a single penny from any of them--nor is it likely at this point I ever will. These days the entire system is rigged toward the large medical groups, pharmaceutical companies, and the medical device manufacturers, because of the tremendous amount of money they have at their disposal.

CHAPTER 33

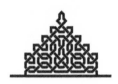

Ted: Beware the Medical-Industrial Complex

There is another way for unscrupulous medical companies and corporations to get money from you that you are not even remotely aware of...and this is what happened to me.

At the time I had absolutely no debt. My home was paid for. I did not have a car loan, although I did not drive a new car either. I held no credit card debt. And I owed no one any money at all. My job was very secure. I had a great boss; one who was such a good guy that he made sure we had not just medical insurance, but that we had the best medical insurance one could get.

My physicians' groups knew that if they used the correct procedure codes matched with the correct diagnosis codes when billing the patient (me), they could literally reach into my insurance "wallet." Their business mode of operation was presumably to use the most profitable procedure codes to match the most profitable diagnosis codes in order to generate the largest monetary return available to them from health insurance companies.

In my case, the doctors simply had to copy my insurance cards and subsequently bill the insurance company hundreds of thousands of dollars without my ever knowing what in fact they were doing. I never even received the actual bills--it was all computerized. The computer programs that were processing these claims were completely automated. That means no human oversight was done to make sure that what was being done was actually benefiting the patient.

Had I not had such good insurance--had I not held a card that could gain them access to millions of dollars in benefits (by knowing the right codes)--there would have been no "disability" attached to me, the person that I am now. Instead, I might have had a just a simple back problem that flared up now and again, like so many other humans have.

I might have had a problem in my ankle...but it turned out to be related to something completely different than what was diagnosed.

Take a look at the photo following this page.

This photo depicts the growth on my lower left leg just below my knee. It was pressing on the main nerve that ran down my leg. This was the reason for the pain I had in my ankle.

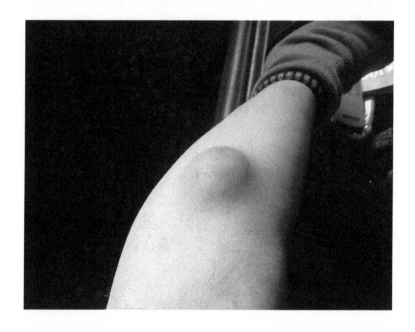

This pain had nothing to do with what was identified and was instead billed as "Spondylolisthesis." This "made-up abnormality" is thought to occur in a large portion of the human population by some human genome researchers. Some people, as in my case, have what is considered to be a mild case, meaning the placement of the vertebrae most likely will not cause any major problems. In fact, some researchers determined that this condition is triggered in the fetus by

Ben Dales and B. B. Beaudreaux

leftover genes that were turned on because humans evolved to walk upright extremely quickly, in terms of evolution. Consequently, these researchers determined that the vertebrae was really in the correct position, and actually left over from when humans were not using solely an upright gait.

Some geneticists believe that this congenital condition is a remnant of when we humans were "walking on all fours," a period in our evolution when the bones in the spine were not supposed to be aligned up and down, or vertically. They were instead aligned back and forth, or horizontally. This did make the case for what pain management doctors called a pinched nerve, but that was a complete misnomer. Pinched nerves have nothing to do with Spondylolisthesis. If you have ever had a real pinched nerve, then you realize it could have only been caused by trauma--a car accident or a fall from a cliff or being hit by a baseball bat in the back--but not because it just happened to be the way you were born.

So how did they get the money from me?

They got it simply by knowing which diagnosis codes were insurance-approved and Medicare-approved. They matched those with approved procedure codes and processed them electronically through the automated billing process. This increased the finances of the "pain management" doctors and other physicians' groups, both of whom were in the business of increasing the bottom line to corporate entities issuing stock to stockholders in order to become extremely lucrative.

It was the million dollar code--and just by pairing the correct diagnosis and procedure codes, they opened the safe. In fact they not only opened it, but indeed they found a safe that kept giving and giving and giving, more and more money every single time they "opened" it.

Every time I stepped into a doctor's office, the routine was the same. The first inquiry, even before my name--and yes, even before "Do you need assistance?" was "I need to see your insurance card and your ID." Many physician groups and hospitals will not even admit you if you do not have a valid insurance card.

If you say "I don't have insurance," they cannot help you (and they don't want to). Why? It's because then they would have to bill you directly. And then they would have to reveal to you the outrageous amounts they are charging you for a simple bandage or an aspirin.

When I was introduced to the SAN Medical Device Company mini-neurostimulator, it was on the condition that it had to be pre-approved

Ben Dales and B. B. Beaudreaux

by my insurance company before it could even be discussed with me by the representatives from SAN Medical Device Company and by my doctor. I was required to have a letter (actually, two letters) of approval--showing that this device had been "pre-approved." I had to have the letters in hand before they would even talk to me about what this device was supposed to do and how it was alleged to work.

My insurance company did in fact approve the surgery, but ironically, someone hadn't filed the approval letter properly. The matching of the proper codes spit out a rejection letter. Four weeks after the neurostimulator surgery, I received a "bill the patient directly" invoice from the hospital requesting the amount of $103,000. Had I myself not kept copies of those misfiled pre-approval letters, I would have been on the hook for the total amount.

When the correct billing procedure was later used, the charge was reduced to a "mere" $53,000--negotiated and paid for by my insurance.

Investing in the Medical Device Industry

Have you looked to see what exactly is in your stock portfolio? If you ask for a breakdown from your financial planner, you will see the exact companies that you are investing in. I am sure you will find huge pharmaceutical companies along with medical device manufacturers. You will also likely find health insurance companies and corporations that have no bearing to what they actually are, what they're developing, or what they represent.

They're likely the companies that are making stockholders quite wealthy. Health is big business.

But here's the thing--by investing in the companies that do not ethically test devices and procedures, you're also contributing to the process that destroys people's lives.

I know this because I had the very stock in my retirement account that led to my disability.

When I had money in these types of investments, I was happy at the time. I was getting a return. But after digging deeper, I realized I had been investing in my own demise.

CHAPTER 34

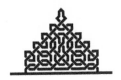

Deni: Playing the Game

Ted and I both recall the day we received the outrageous bill of more than $103,000 for the implant of the SAN mini-neurostimulator. It showed that our insurance had denied coverage and thus refused payment of any portion of this amount. This bill carefully identified the acceptable forms of payment to be used.

And the payment was expected right away.

I often reflect back to the "old-school" days when paying for all things medical was so much simpler. A doctor's appointment typically meant a $5 or $10 copayment at most. Surgeries were often covered in full, even if there were some extraneous charges that trickled in during the later weeks. It seemed that charges were calculated correctly, for the most part, the first time. There was usually little need to follow up with phone calls questioning the patient portion amounts expected.

This invoice of more than $103,000 of course required a lot of follow-up, both with the hospital asking for its money and with our insurance carrier denying the claim. We went back and forth with phone calls to and from both until the insurance company finally told us the reason for the denial: the surgery performed had never been pre-approved.

We knew that was not true. Not only had we received a letter from the insurance company itself showing the surgery was pre-approved, but also we had given a copy of this very letter to the hospital's billing department before the surgery was performed.

Why would the insurance company itself deny a claim for a surgical procedure it had already approved?

Why would the hospital send us an outrageous billing amount based on the insurance denial when it already had a copy of the letter showing just the opposite?

What would have happened had we not kept our own copy of the approval letter in a file ready to produce? Would we have been liable for more than $103,000 on our own?

Finally, what is really going on behind the scenes with health insurance companies--and with hospitals--that they do not bat an eye or offer even the slightest acknowledgment that they really goofed this one up? Do these businesses even know or much less care that this is now the norm?

Yes, they certainly are businesses.

The point is that through the oft-painful experience of handling billing invoices that arrive in the mail with all kinds of errors, oversights, undersights, and the like, we as patient consumer advocates are forced to "pay or play." By that I mean we have the choice of just paying the bill as it arrives (which is what the insurance companies want), or we can delve into playing the game of billing and coding by contacting the insurance as well as the service provider and going from there. Each time is a new experience, often a new challenge, and in most cases, an uninvited new lesson to learn.

In this day and age, these types of situations happen so frequently that patients often are not surprised when they occur. It seems so absurd that this has become the norm that we jokingly wonder aloud if these companies are giving out bonuses or other incentives for employees who allow such mistakes to happen.

One friend of ours works for the health benefits department of one of the largest employers in Chicago. Her good friend was hired and went through the training for a dental health insurance company. This insurance employee revealed that part of the training involved "competence at being incompetent." The expectation was that one out of every ten patient claims received was to be "lost" or "misplaced" or should otherwise just "disappear." This allowed the dental company to receive higher payments directly from the patients, at least from those not bothering to dispute their billed amounts.

It is certainly understandable that if 10% of all claims are delayed or otherwise non-existent, it could and would affect the company's bottom-line favorably, to say the least. It makes one wonder how many of these bills are not disputed? How many are blindly paid by unsuspecting patients?

CHAPTER 35

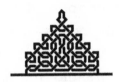

Deni: Remember when doctors were in it to save lives?

This may be considered "old-school," but there was a time when bright, energetic young men and women studied medicine in order to make a difference. It was the prospect of saving lives, of helping keep people healthy, and of guiding these very patients throughout their lifetimes in caring ways. These very patients became family friends of the doctor. Hence, the commonly-used term "family doctor." Conversely, the doctor was a friend of the family. Back in the now-revered Fifties, it was the norm for doctors to make house calls if needed. It was not unusual, either. It was expected.

I suppose there are doctors around like that today in these modern times, but it is certainly not the norm. Ask a few people some questions about their doctor...or more likely, their doctors. In former times, people tended to go to one doctor for everything. We all know that is no longer the case. People tend to have more than one doctor, and most have several doctors--one for each current affliction. This may or may not work to the benefit of us patients. We are told that since we are seeing specialists for each affliction, we are receiving more specialized treatment. A drawback here, however, is that one doctor may not necessarily know what another is prescribing or how they are treating said patient.

Nevertheless, the existence of multiple doctors for multiple purposes does work to the benefit of doctors, to the benefit of medical insurance companies, and to the benefit of prescription drug companies. For one thing, it has increased the monetary intake collectively of all these entities. It has raised the financial bar of each one. Instead of one invoice charge to the patient from one doctor for an appointment with multiple purposes, there are now multiple invoices to the patient from as many doctors (or more) as there are purposes. Insurance coverage now extends to all such doctors and their purposes. Because insurance companies have many more doctors to contract, they are able to charge increasing amounts annually to patients for coverage. Prescription drug companies both

Ben Dales and B. B. Beaudreaux

subsequently and consequently receive more prescription orders, since more doctors are in practice to prescribe them.

At this point, it is appropriate to pause for a small yet significant sidebar. The previous paragraph's last two sentences contained the words "treatment" and "treat." It is worthwhile to delve into the dictionary definitions of these words. Concerning the latter in terms of traditional medical usage, "treat" is defined in Webster's as "to care for or to deal with medically or surgically." Concerning the former in the same light, "treatment" is defined in Webster's as "a substance or technique used in treating." Both definitions represent long-held usage practices in the medical field; e.g., "In order to treat his patient, the doctor dictated a treatment plan."

Currently, one can allude to alternate meanings of treat and treatment. These alternate meanings are certainly not recognized nor admitted by doctors and their staff, but a case may be made of these meanings just the same.

Upon first entering or even contacting a doctor's office, an initial question is "What is your insurance?"

This question is posed long before it is actually needed, such as at the time of billing and not at the earlier time of treatment. One of perhaps multiple reasons for posing the insurance question so early just might be that the doctor and his staff can learn what "treats" await them in the patient's insurance. They can learn early what their resulting "treatment" may be from that insurance, as they plan and devise the many ways they can "treat" themselves to a patient's insurance benefits. Doctor and staff become well-versed and downright knowledgeable about what is offered by each of the many insurance options, which insurances cover and cover well (not to mention, pay well) for which specified treatments the doctor may wish to prescribe (or not prescribe, in the case of a patient having "low-cost basic insurance" and/or a patient being underinsured).

This is an entirely new concept of "treatment" and "being treated" in the medical field. The question, however, now becomes who is being treated to what? Is it not possible the patient's dictated treatment is currently driven by insurance coverage and allowances that serve to "treat" the doctor for having prescribed them?

One might pause at this point to ask for proof of these types of contentions about what treatment is, and what and who is actually the driving force behind the treatments being dictated. It turns out there is plenty of proof.

Ben Dales and B. B. Beaudreaux

One example involves the pacemaker as a prescribed treatment for heart problems. The history of this medical device is detailed quite well by author Katy Butler and her book, *Knocking On Heaven's Door*. In the chapter entitled "The Business of Lifesaving," she traces the existence of the very first pacemaker implanted as happening in 1958. She goes on to write that within two years, "the pacemaker moved...onto small assembly lines." She states that the first pacemaker company...by the end of December 1960, "had taken orders for fifty pacemakers, priced at $375 each."

Our author acknowledges, "Sales were slow at first. In 1962, Medtronic lost $144,000." The following year, it "sold only twelve hundred pacemakers and edged barely into the black." It was at this time that "the Arthur D. Little consulting company estimated that only ten thousand people worldwide would ever need pacemakers." This all changed shortly, when "in 1965, Medicare... was established...and approved the pacemaker for reimbursement the following year for any American over the age of sixty-five with a medical need for one."

Whether pacemakers were needed or not, they began to be prescribed by doctors who now knew that prescribing them would bring in the money. "In the first full year of Medicare reimbursement...

Medtronic sold 7,400 pacemakers, six times as many as it had three years before...and made a profit of nearly $308,000." By 1968, "it reported annual sales of $10 million and profits of more than $1 million." By 1970, this company's "annual sales had more than doubled, to $22 million. Pacemakers had become the company's cash cow." Of course each pacemaker implant brought in revenue to the doctors who did the surgical implants and to the prescription drug companies supplying the necessary prescription drugs.

It is a clear illustration that Medicare offered many more options for "treatment" to those doctors and prescription companies for dictating the treatment of a pacemaker.

Author Katy Butler goes on to report a similar story with another company. The initial product was the heart valve, another example of a medical device whose usage also increased exponentially after becoming Medicare-approved. Millions of dollars were generated, going straight into the pockets of the medical device company and later of similar companies, along with the doctors who inserted them surgically, as well as hospitals and prescription drug companies.

The floodgates now opened, scads of new medical devices were proposed, created, and tried in attempts to secure that ever-precious Medicare

Ben Dales and B. B. Beaudreaux

approval for usage. The path leading to this almost always included paid peer reviews (often by doctors who would eventually be prescribing them) and monetary and other bonuses to doctors who did in fact prescribe them, before and after Medicare approval.

It is noteworthy here to mention that not all such devices were success stories. Two of these non-success stories were the bone growth stimulator and the mini-neurostimulator.

CHAPTER 36

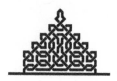

Ted: My Health Insurance Survey

A thousand dollars was a lot of money for me at the time, but I wanted to gather some unbiased answers from the public about health insurance. I decided to create a survey and go back to Chicago, as it was the closest cosmopolitan city where I could "stage" this survey. I had considered Detroit due to its being the largest city in my state of residence. However, Detroit is just a tunnel ride away from Canada. I might have ended up with a lot of answers that were from Canadians who all have affordable health insurance through their own government.

It was strange to me at the time that our northern neighbor Canada would have such a well-functioning health care system, although I had known for years that buying medications from

Ben Dales and B. B. Beaudreaux

Canada was a real money-saver. In fact, after I became disabled, many people I met who were not insured had no choice but to buy their medicines from Canada. As a result, there was much blowback about this practice by pharmaceutical companies as serious questions were raised about the "potency and grade" of the pharmaceuticals coming across the border. This was equally true for people who were going to Mexico, not only to obtain their needed medications, but also to have everything from medical procedures and tests to dental work. In fact, the term "medical tourism" was and is being used by many people who are going out of the U.S. for elective surgeries and other medical procedures. Some people are even traveling all the way to Indonesia because the lowered costs of procedures there would not only pay for the trip, but the follow-up care and recovery tally up to be just a fraction of what the same surgery in the U.S. would be.

That is why this questionnaire of mine was so vital to my understanding of why people in the U.S. have health insurance premiums that are exorbitantly expensive.

Now, I had planned to use a thousand dollars for offering free ten-dollar lunches with gift cards that could be used at a popular eatery with multiple locations in Chicago's Loop. As it turned out, when

I went to purchase the gift cards, the individual menu items were each at least $10 - and that was "a la carte." With dismay, I ended up making the gift cards $15 dollars each. This is because I had the feeling that people would not even stop to answer the three questions I had posed for them for just half of the cost of a lunch. So, an expense of $1500 was what I had to pay. I also knew that I would get a few homeless people who maybe didn't have jobs and would just want the card in order to eat, but my target group was people in the workforce.

My best chance to find people interested in earning a free lunch by answering my queries was, as one might expect, to approach working persons on their way to their jobs in the morning. I also knew that homeless people who wanted to answer or take the survey were going to approach me. Although my main target group was working people, I could not deny anyone the chance for a free lunch, because it wouldn't have been fair. And by fair, I mean it wouldn't have been fair to the study, and it wouldn't have been fair to the homeless who (as has been pointed out by many) became homeless usually through no fault of their own. In fact, many had become homeless because of the exact thing I wanted people to know about--medical issues. Some found themselves homeless because of their own medical issues, and some because of medical issues from members of their

Ben Dales and B. B. Beaudreaux

own family or because of an illness of someone they loved, or, sadly, had lost.

So, bright and very early on a warm Thursday morning in the spring, I had Deni plop me down on the corner of Randolph and Michigan with a sign that read, "FREE LUNCH - JUST ANSWER THREE QUICK QUESTIONS!" While making the sign, I also added a parenthetical phrase that stated, "$15 Gift Card Redeemable for a Free Lunch," because as was pointed out to me by a colleague, many people think there is no such thing as a free lunch, as the saying goes.

So there I was with my clipboards packed, the numbered questionnaire forms, and a stack of $15 gift cards in my pocket. I set up a tall, narrow table to write on, positioned in a rather inconspicuous corner of the Chicago Cultural Center.

As the first few minutes of my day progressed, I realized I had to be a little proactive by asking people if they would like a gift card for a free lunch. Many people didn't answer back until finally a young woman looked at me as I smiled, and she said, "Sure, I'll answer your three questions."

As the morning progressed and more people were on their way to work, the pace of "surveying the public" with my three questions picked up rapidly.

The first one was simple: "Do you have health insurance?"

The second query was based on how they answered the first question. If the person answered "Yes," then I would continue with: "And, why do you have health insurance?"

If the answer was, "No, I do not have health insurance," my next question would be, "If you could have health insurance, would you take it and why?"

This would cover both scenarios to learn what the person thought about why people have health insurance.

Now, the third question's answer was what I was really after in the survey.

This third question was at the crux of the issue I was trying to determine for my book. It actually had very little bearing on the first two questions. It was just that in order to get realistic answers to the third question, the first two had to be asked in order to properly set up the third and final question.

So, without any bearing on how the first two questions were answered, the final question was:

"And, why is there health insurance?"

By 9:30 a.m. I had a stack of completed questionnaires. As I figured, almost all of my participants answered the questions the exact way I thought they would. For example, looking back to the first woman, the survey went as such:

"Do you have health insurance?"

"Yes, I do," she replied.

"Why do you have health insurance?"

"In case I get sick."

"Why is there health insurance?"

"In case I get sick," she replied again.

And so the the morning rolled by with almost everyone en route to work answering essentially the same way.

There were two people, one a man and one a woman, who both said, "No, I do not have health insurance."

Of course the second question was then rephrased, and predictably, they both said, "Yes, I would have health insurance to protect me."

Then the final question came out as all the rest: "Why is there health insurance?"

They both replied, "In case I were to get in an accident or in case I become ill."

The next passerby was a well-dressed man, probably in his late fifties. He was just meandering his way up Michigan Avenue in no big hurry.

I knew that in order to complete my 100 "case questions," I would need to be a little more persistent in asking. I therefore said in a rather loud voice, "Sir, I'm almost done with my survey. I have only a few more people to ask my three questions. Would you please help me finish?"

He read my sign and then quietly replied, "I really don't need your gift card."

I said, "That's okay. I just need a couple more people, then I can wrap up everything. Really, sir, it will just take less than thirty seconds of your time and I really need to finish this project. Please, sir, I just need a few more people."

Now I don't know if he took pity on me because I had my handle walker next to the table with the clipboard and pens, or if he just thought he would be doing a good deed for the day, but he approached and said, "Sure, I'll answer your three questions."

Ben Dales and B. B. Beaudreaux

"Okay, thank you very much, sir. I truly appreciate your help. Now the first question is: 'Do you have health insurance?'"

"Absolutely!" He replied with a smile.

"Great," I said. "The second question is: 'Why do you have health insurance?'"

His eyebrows raised and his lips kind of puckered a bit.

"Well, I tell you, my friend, if something horrible would happen, or in the event that a catastrophic injury or illness befalls me, I have health insurance so I wouldn't have to surrender my assets to cover my medical bills. Or in the event that it were truly a matter of life or death, I have health insurance so I would never become bankrupt by having to have major medical assistance from a hospital or a physician or a myriad of other medical professionals who are trained to keep people from dying. Actually, I like to think that it is a kind of service offered to the public."

As I scurried to scribble down his lengthy comment, it struck me that this was the first person who actually gave me an answer other than "In case I get sick."

I started thinking that this man is really intelligent, or….

"That's a great response," I replied. "Thank you for your honesty and clarity. I wish all the people before you would have been so forthright when answering. So, I have the third question for you, and then I would like you to have our free lunch card."

Even though he had previously declined the free lunch card, his reply nonetheless startled me a bit. This is because he was the first to express these very sentiments to me.

His reply was, "No, that's alright, my friend. I do not need the card. You keep the card and have a nice lunch for yourself after all your surveying. I know you must have gotten up really early today to get this done. Doing surveys off the street is tedious, and I'm sure you've encountered many people who thought you were out to sell them something."

"Thank you, sir. That is very generous of you."

Again, I was startled by his amazing insight as to what I had gone through all morning. It was almost as if he had been watching me or listening to all the people participating in this survey.

"I still have one more question. Why is there health insurance?"

Ben Dales and B. B. Beaudreaux

He hesitated only briefly. Without blinking an eye, he responded: "Well, as I said, I like to think of it as a service we are providing to the public so that if something unexpected happens to them, they will not be financially ruined in case of illness or accident."

Hmm, I think I might know where this is going.

Playing naive, I said, "Oh, I see. It's kind of like a wager. People pay into a pool of money, and it's there for them if they need it later, right?"

"Well, partially," he admitted. "But you must understand that insurance of all types does not come from solely philanthropic institutions. These are corporations...and all corporations exist, at least initially, to earn a return on an initial investment. If the company grows and there is a demand or an ability to extend market shares, the company offers stock to provide a means of financial investment to more people and a way to grow internally and offer more services to customers."

I almost fell over.

"You know sir, you are the first person out of 90-some people that I questioned this morning who actually gave me that answer, and I personally believe that is the most correct answer for the third question. You were the only person out of all the people I asked who did not respond with, 'Health insurance exists in case I get sick,' or something to that effect. You truly are a very knowledgeable man. Do you mind if I ask you one more question?"

"Not at all, I'd be happy to answer."

"What do you do for a living?"

With a big smile and a bit of a chuckle, he replied, "I have to know all about these things, as an executive of one of the largest insurance providers in the U.S."

"An executive? In what capacity?" I asked.

He hesitated, possibly realizing I was probing too far.

"Let's just say I keep track of the pool of money to ensure that more money comes in than goes out."

At this point I realized he was not going to be forthcoming with any further queries, so I just said to him, "Well, thank you. Are you sure you don't want your gift card?"

He rolled out a big laugh and said, "No, my friend, you give it to someone who is really hungry."

"Thank you, sir. Thank you very, very much," I said as he turned to walk away.

"You're welcome, and you take care of yourself. I hope you got what you need."

If he only knew! The only person that truly realized why health insurance companies exist at all was an executive of one of the most recognizable health insurance companies in the world. He knew the right answer because of his job position. He knew it was all about making money. He was the only one--well, the only one out of all my participants.

By this time, the street was almost clear of pedestrians. I still had a few gift cards left to hand out, but I was extremely tired, and the prospects for another person answering my questionnaire were low.

Then from somewhere behind me, I heard a gruff voice: "I'll answer your three questions."

This man sounded like Kramer from Seinfeld. As I turned around, he even kind of reminded me of Kramer, only he was dressed very shabbily and I guessed at once he was homeless.

"Okay, sir," I began, "I want to ask you if you have health insurance?"

"Hell no. Does it look like I have health insurance?"

"Well, no, sir, but I'm not trying to be sarcastic, it's just that these are the three questions."

"Well, then ask me the the other two," he demanded.

"Okay, now if you could, would you have health insurance?"

"Hell no!"

Now this really threw me for a loop. Here was this obviously homeless guy and he wouldn't want to have health insurance. Then he pressed on, but on a different level.

"Health insurance, HA!" He scoffed. "You know what health insurance is? You know what they are?"

"What are they?" I asked.

"They're a bunch of thieves! The only reason they exist is to make billionaires out of the founders, and millionaires out of the corporate executives," he ranted. "It's a big scam. They're nothing but con men and swindlers. I wouldn't have health insurance if you paid me to take it."

Ben Dales and B. B. Beaudreaux

Flabbergasted, I took the rest of the stack of gift cards and just handed them to him. He and the executive were the only two people out of everyone I'd asked who truly understood why health insurance companies exist. One, a high-ranking executive making millions from the 99%, and the other, a homeless man who had nothing more in life than his common sense.

CHAPTER 37

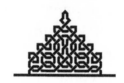

Ted: The Evolution of Health Care

Why do hospitals exist?

Wikipedia reveals a history of hospitals stretching back over 2500 years, from the Ascelpian temples in ancient Greece to the military hospitals in ancient Rome. No civilian hospital existed until the emergence of the Christian period, with the first Christian hospitals appearing toward the end of the 4th century. It was not until the early modern era in the late 1500s when care and healing would transition into a secular affair, or at least become shared with religious hospital institutions.

There is interesting proof found in German language vocabulary that hospitals were strictly religious enterprises. The German word for hospital is Krankenhaus, whose literal translation

Ben Dales and B. B. Beaudreaux

to English would be "Sick House" (indicating the oft-humorous and blunt translation of German words). However, the German word for nurse is Krankenschwester, which translates literally to English as "Sick Sister." The "Sister" here refers to the fact that nurses were not only women, but religious sisters. We are told that dating back to medieval Europe, hospitals were run by and care was given by monks and nuns. Likewise, an old French term for hospital was hotel-Dieu, translating to English as "hostel of God." Many early European hospitals were actually connected to monasteries. According to prevailing religious beliefs of those times, little or no compensation from patients was expected or charged. Care and healing given was instead based on benevolence and charity.

Wikipedia also informs us that the U.S. National Library of Medicine credits the hospital as being a product of medieval Islamic civilization. Islamic hospitals contrasted from their contemporaneous Christian institutions as being more elaborate institutions with a wider range of functions than the Christians' poor and sick relief facilities. Instead of being based upon charity and good works earned in the face of the church, in Islam there was a moral imperative to treat the ill regardless of financial status. Islamic hospitals tended to be large, urban structures and many of them were open to all, whether male or female, civilian or military, child or adult, rich or poor, Muslim or non-Muslim. Finally, Islamic benevolence was not just for hospital care. Islamic hospitals served several purposes: as a center for medical treatment, a home for patients in recovery from illness or accidents, an insane asylum, and a retirement home providing basic maintenance needs for the aged and infirm.

Islamic hospitals were forbidden by law to turn away patients who were unable to pay. Financial support came from various outside sources--part of the state budget went toward maintaining hospitals, plus charitable foundations were formed to support hospitals. Services of the hospitals were free for all citizens, and in fact patients were sometimes even given a small stipend to support recovery upon discharge. Only individual physicians occasionally charged fees.

Suffice it to say, we have come a long way since the days of charity, benevolence, and free hospital care. At some point in the late 1800s, most hospitals largely converted to secular institutions. Non-profit hospitals converted to public hospitals. At some point, at least in the U.S., health care became a for-profit business. Therefore, in this day and age (and country), we get a totally different response

Ben Dales and B. B. Beaudreaux

to the question in the beginning of this chapter.

Ask anyone that question. If you do, you will likely get this answer: "Hospitals exist in case you get sick." You can ask the same question about health insurance companies. Ask those whom you believe to be very intelligent, and they will most likely reply, "Insurance companies make sure you can pay for treatment and care if you get hurt, so you can get back on your feet again."

If only these reasons were true.

The real fact is that today's hospitals exist for one thing and one thing only.

They exist to make money.

The same is true for health insurance companies...or any kind of insurance companies, for that matter. There is no great giving, benevolent institution sanctioned by a supreme being that mandates available services to ensure you don't die if you get hit by a bus. Each of these entities exist primarily to make money for the people who have invested in them.

Hospitals could not exist if they did not make money. In fact, the ones that do not make money are often shuttered and closed down while the buildings and properties are sold to other entities that believe they can turn a profit by providing better medical services to patients with medical needs. Even hospitals that are run by the government need to make a profit in order to pay the people working there. It's a simple fact of life that if you want to live your life in the U.S. after getting sick, it is going to cost you money.

Insurance used to be the "hedge bet" against catastrophes that might occur to one or to one's family. According to Wikipedia, this country's first health insurance policies date back to Civil War times and only offered coverage against accidents from travel by rail or steamboat. The process was simple enough; one wouldn't lose everything worked for in order to ensure that loved ones would survive.

However, at some point back in the Sixties that idea became extinct. With the onset of Medicare in 1966, new insurance companies were popping up all over the place. This was largely because the existing ones were making a fortune for the people that founded them. It was a simple bet that people (insurance customers) would more likely die than need medical care costing more than the amount they paid into their insurance premiums over their lifetime. It was a hedge bet coming out in favor of insurance companies a majority of the time.

As time went on, though, technology became increasingly successful at changing the human

Ben Dales and B. B. Beaudreaux

condition. More and more people were able to survive accidents and sudden illnesses or other maladies due to advances in medical research. The result? It put a severe hit on the profits being made by medical insurance companies and hospitals.

The outcome?

Well, that is easily understood by anyone who has ever paid even one medical insurance premium. This is borne out in statistics as well, available from many sources. Per capita, U.S health care expenditures increased from an annual $147 in 1960 to $8,402 in 2010. Likewise, health care spending as a percentage of U.S. Gross Domestic Product (GDP) was a mere 5.2% in 1960 compared to 17.9% in 2010.

Is this becoming a trend? For your answer, you only need to fast forward two or three years. This is documented quite early (p. 13) in Jeanne Lenzer's book, The Danger Within Us, when she writes: Healthcare is now the single biggest sector of the U.S. economy. It is bigger than big oil, bigger than big banking, and bigger even than the famous military-industrial complex that President Dwight Eisenhower warned about in his farewell speech. In 2013, the most generous estimate pegged the price of the military-industrial complex at $1.3

trillion, while healthcare expenditures in 2015 were $3.2 trillion, consuming nearly one of every five dollars spent in the U.S.

And of course, the beat goes on....

CHAPTER 38

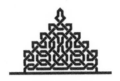

Ted: The Coding and Billing Game

The new pain management clinics you see and hear about on television and radio do not primarily exist to help patients control the pain they are experiencing. Instead, the various groups of anesthesiologists who organized together to start up these new mega money-making businesses saw a huge opportunity to make tremendous amounts of money. The opportunity window opened up to them, because Medicare-approved steroidal epidural injections to people on Medicare. When a person in pain goes into one of these clinics or even tries just to make an appointment, many times this person is immediately told, "All we do is give shots."

In my case, after moving from the city to the country, one of the first steps I took was contacting all the pain clinics within a hundred-mile radius. Without even knowing my medical history, the receptionists on staff (that is, if you could even get through to an actual person) were trained to say the phrase, "All we do is give shots."

My constant first thought in each case was, How ignorant is that opening statement for a pain management clinic to be using? Shouldn't the first concern be understanding what is being experienced by the patient and then administering the appropriate pain remediation?

I have come to understand that medical systems have not evolved to help people. They exist (and yes, exist as giant enterprises) for the primary purpose of **making money**. They do not necessarily make this money directly from patients--in fact, they do not bill the patients except for the relatively small copays. Behind the scenes, so to speak, these enterprises are adept at using the proper diagnosis codes along with the corresponding procedure codes for filing to the patient's medical insurance or Medicare. Before the onset of computers, and before the computer algorithms became so complex, medical offices used to reveal to patients the actual cost of doctor visits and clinical or hospital lab procedures. Now with the advancement of computer science and with billing and coding, the only information that patients are allowed to know is what the deductible is and what the copay is. This is exactly the way that all the people who are making money from the medical industry want it to be and how they want it to continue. If patients really knew the amounts being billed, they would question each specific treatment or procedure and its alleged cost.

Fortunately, transparency is being mandated by Congress which requires hospitals to itemize each specific charge in detail, with the same mandate for clinics and doctor's offices. It remains to be seen just how much detail these entities will get away with revealing and not revealing.

From my experience and research, I've learned that the insurance companies and Medicare do not regularly review the charges, or at least they are not actually individually reviewed by a staff person. As long as the procedure code matches the diagnosis code, the computers are programmed to allow the bill to pass through the program, and for a credit amount or figure to be sent to the providers' database field. Then when all the claims are processed, that total credit is issued to the account of that service provider.

This is why so much fraud is able to occur through Medicare by deceptive medical providers. No one person ever checks to see who is getting paid what (unless it is the savvy, curious patient calling to check on a questionable invoice amount). This current system of programmed accountability keeps it all the more simple for the many people utilizing this mega medical system, which is automated.

If there is a wrong procedure code assigned to a diagnosis code, you, as the patient, do know it right away upon receiving the bill. This is likely because the claim has been rejected and in turn, you get billed some enormous amount. You are not being billed the negotiated rate that the "execs" have worked out with Medicare or with medical insurance companies. You are instead billed for the "pie-in-the-sky" amount they have come up with in their billing process.

Ben Dales and B. B. Beaudreaux

CHAPTER 39

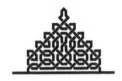

Deni: The Coding Levels

Coding and Billing - Level One

The current system of coding and billing is complicated. There are diagnosis codes and there are procedure codes, and the list of thousands of billing codes keeps growing bigger and bigger. It was overheard that the system has become so complicated that there is now a separate billing code to use for treatment of individuals specifically injured on a Ski-Doo jet ski while on Lake Michigan.

Several times I have been told by my insurance carrier that I need to advise my medical service provider to resubmit the claim with a different code, because the original one submitted was not being covered correctly. This has happened to me so many times that now I almost expect the request for every medical procedure or visit will require follow-up.

Every time, the routine is the same. I receive an Explanation Of Benefits (EOB) from the insurance company, which itself is written with so many codes, abbreviations, and apparently internal code words that it takes me awhile just to understand it. In any case, the calculated amount for "Patient Responsibility" is higher (often much higher) than it is supposed to be, according to what my medical insurance card states (4%). I then must phone the insurance company, going through a series of automated voicemail prompts that easily takes up ten minutes. I finally get through to a "customer representative" who more often than not puts me on hold for an indeterminate length of time ("Please hold one moment while I check"), only to come back to me apologetically to announce that I must be transferred to someone else.

Here comes another indeterminate time of being in the "Land of Hold." Of course, it would not be so bad if the hold music were not so "elevator." I once suggested seriously that hold music should at least be fun and somewhat tongue-in-cheek. I'd like to hear "I'm Sorry" by Brenda Lee, "Tired of Waiting" by The Kinks, "Hold On, I'm Coming" by Sam and Dave, "Hold Me, Hold Me; Never Let Me Go" by Mel Carter, etcetera, etcetera, you get the idea. At least one could enjoy being in the proverbial "Land of Hold!"

Ben Dales and B. B. Beaudreaux

Eventually I do get through to someone who may--or may not--be able to help me. I am almost always told to contact my service provider to request the bill be resubmitted with a different and more correct coding. After so many phone calls like this over and over, I can share one ready fact of feeling. I feel as if I am doing the work for both companies.

I have learned a few things from so many calls like this. When told to call my service provider, I now convey that I will not be the go-between messenger. ("However, I will gladly be placed on hold while you call them on my behalf. Do you need the phone number, or do you already have it?") I take copious notes about what I'm told by whom by name ("Spell that for me, please") and at what time on what date. This is because far too often on these callbacks I am asked, "On what date did you call?" and "What was the name of the person who told you that?" I am ready to fire back with all the specifics, more than I am asked. This, I have learned, produces results--at least as far as the phone call I'm currently on is concerned.

Yes, I have been forced to begin learning how to play the coding game. I now ask each representative who mentions coding just what code was used, as opposed to what code should be used. I am compiling my own list as I go and as it relates to our lives and our treatments. Since we do not plan to jet ski on a Ski-Doo on Lake Michigan, I do not need that code in my list.

Coding and Billing - Level Two

I can now proudly (if not painfully) say that I continue to "level up" in my expertise of coding as it is related to billing. With each insurance challenge that appears, I find myself deeper into this million-dollar game.

One such challenge happened as a result of my annual physical check-up that I have received for more than three decades--ever since my father died unexpectedly at age 56 when I was only 35. On at least two occasions over the years, my annual physical has served to prevent a couple of instances of potentially serious and life-threatening diseases for me.

Excepting the copay, my insurance has always covered in full one physical per year. A recent annual physical happened in December, long after my yearly deductible had been met, yet still within the same calendar year during which I had received no such physical. As usual, the billing statement arrived a few months later--in the new year. It was quite a bit higher than it seemed it should be.

Ben Dales and B. B. Beaudreaux

My first step is always to locate in my files the Explanation of Benefits (EOB) statement previously received from my insurance carrier. I located this particular EOB and recalled that when first seeing it, I thought it might be error-ridden. I did not pursue it at the time, as it was confusing to me and frankly, did not require payment yet. This is something else I have learned in my "journey," not to panic or become frantic until necessary-- which means not until the actual billing invoice arrives. Otherwise, one runs the risk of making all the needed follow-up phone calls twice. Plus, trying to solve the problem early, i.e., before it is a "problem" bill, likely means having to pay earlier than I would with normal billing time period procedures.

As it turned out, the EOB appeared not to have paid anything at all. Upon pursuing this by phone with my insurance carrier, I was told it was true--that nothing was covered. I countered with the fact that this was my annual physical, something that has always been covered. The representative quickly informed me that is no longer the case with an actual physical; what is in fact covered is an annual "wellness visit." Apart from being initially incredulous, I asked what was the difference between an annual physical and an annual wellness visit. The representative could neither answer this nor find any information about the difference for me. I was referred to my doctor's office for the answer. I knew I would have to phone there anyway, following this surprising revelation.

Not only did I phone, but I happened to have another new appointment with this doctor since this was a few months after my physical. He chuckled as he told me there was absolutely no difference in the procedures, that it was just semantics being used by the insurance company. He promised to look into it right away and have it fixed, so that the bill would be reworked and rebilled.

Funny thing is, later on I happened to share my doctor's verbiage ("it is just semantics") both with representatives from my insurance and with a billing representative for this doctor's own billing network--who laughed and ridiculed the idea that a physical and a wellness visit are the same thing. When I asked them why they would ridicule a physician's summation, they had no logical explanation other than that's the way it was now.

Another "new" incident in billing happened with this same doctor's office. It was based upon a simple office visit bill, which normally does not incur a patient portion payment of even $10. This bill was substantially higher, so I questioned this doctor's office about it. This was another instance of bantering back and forth, only to learn that this

Ben Dales and B. B. Beaudreaux

billing department's computers had listed only the first part of the name of my insurance instead of its full name. This is when I learned that, even though the doctor's treatment and patient procedure may be exactly the same, it can all be billed at higher dollar amounts for "private business" insurance such as BCBS instead of for "public" insurance such as BCBS Medicare Advantage.

Are we starting to feel these "games" that are constantly being played upon us, and at our expense?

Coding and Billing - Level Three

My elevation from Level Two up to Level Three of our ongoing and ever-present game happened as a result of an unfortunate, unforeseen, and eventually unfair incident that occurred with one of the largest pain management clinics in Michigan.

The set-up at this particular clinic was a bit unsettling to us regarding its procedures. Ted was only "allowed" an actual face-to-face consultation visit with his doctor there just once per year. This was in spite of the fact that he was required to have appointments there every three months in order to have his prescriptions written by this clinic. Most of the time, he was only allowed to see the P.A., who had some training, but who had not received enough formal education to be a fully licensed regular doctor. This P.A. in particular was known to be a bit rigid, if not arrogant, and certainly lived up to that image with us.

Early in our relationship with this clinic, Ted was explaining his medical history and especially the experiences that led to his disabled condition and chronic pain. This naturally involved an explanation of the first surgery's failed bone growth stimulator and the subsequent failed SAN Medical Device Company mini-neurostimulator, both of which were large contributors to his disability. As this conversation ensued, I interjected the fact that the irony is the SAN Medical Device Company was an outgrowth of TREND Electronic Medical Device Manufacturers, the company that produced the first device.

"That's not true," insisted the P.A.

I was a bit taken aback by this outburst and denial.

"You might wish to double check that; I've read about it from multiple sources." I pressed on, "Most recently, in *Knocking on Heaven's Door* by Katy Butler. It is right in Chapter 12."

"Oh no. I'm sure of my facts."

We were both a bit miffed by her bedside manner, although we made no further fuss about it.

Toward the end of the first year with this clinic, we at long last were scheduled for the "once per year" face-to-face consultation with our actual doctor there. It was a cordial meeting; the doctor was much more approachable than the P.A. had been with us. However, we had maybe little more than five minutes of actual consultation time during our rather rushed visit, which was full of interruptions. This was solely due to the fact that the office computer system was being transitioned to a brand-new one, and there seemed to be a myriad of problems going on as a result.

Most of our appointment was spent observing the problems encountered by the doctor as he was attempting to send Ted's prescriptions to the local pharmacy via this new computer system. Ted, with his extensive professional background in computers, ended up helping the doctor troubleshoot and trying to solve the transmission problems. An in-house computer technician also entered the foray during our twenty-five minutes to assist.

While all was transpiring before us, I wryly commented that the prescription could have been handwritten by now and we would be at the pharmacy. The humor eased the stress and tension in the room. Eventually, they did succeed in the electronic transmission of the prescriptions, even though it took up more than twenty minutes of our precious annual consultation time with the doctor.

The next annual appointment with the doctor was supposed to occur by the following year's end. The office was not able to accommodate this, so the appointment was made for early January instead (to which we agreed).

However, there was an appointment scheduled anyway for the last week of December, presumably for us to meet with the doctor within the year's time. There was only one problem with this--we were not advised of this December 28 appointment. In fact, we did not even learn about it until just a couple of days prior to our scheduled January appointment, when we received a letter admonishing us for being a no-show and financially charging us for the appointment. The letter also stated that any future such no-show incident could result in our being discharged from this office's and doctor's practice.

We immediately placed a phone call to the doctor's office for clarification and to set the record straight. We questioned why we were being sent such a letter when we had no knowledge whatsoever of the intended appointment. To prove this point,

Ben Dales and B. B. Beaudreaux

we had the receptionist confirm our actual known appointment for the first week of January. She readily did this, which prompted our question, "Why would there even be an appointment in the books and on our written appointment card if we were supposed to be there just the week before in December?"

We brought all our "proof" with us to the January appointment and were thus told that the accused misdeed of being a no-show was being removed from our file. There was also a weak apology, but not one nearly sufficient enough to counter the strong language and actions threatened by the letter we were mailed. Ironically, as it turned out, we did not see the doctor during our January appointment. Once again, we were only able to meet with the P.A.

The next appointment was the one for meeting with the actual doctor and fulfilling the "once per year" commitment. This was to be only our second-ever meeting with our doctor, even though we had been coming to this clinic since the end of the prior year. This appointment was extremely positive and resulted in this doctor dictating a changed course of treatment, which was to be an increase in dosage of pain breakthrough medication.

Upon hearing what Ted was currently taking for pain, his exact words were: "That's really not very much. I am going to increase the prescribed amount."

This appointment concluded with the doctor advising Ted to await the nurse with the prescription. We thanked him for his time, consideration, and understanding of Ted's condition. We also acknowledged to him what a positive experience the appointment had been. While we waited alone in the room, we reflected on how good it was finally to meet with the actual doctor. At some point, a nurse entered with the prescription, which had a lowered dosage amount than what the doctor had just prescribed.

"The doctor himself just authorized an increase," Ted informed her. "Can you please double-check?"

When the nurse returned, she told us the P.A. had changed the course of treatment to a lower dosage.

"Was the doctor aware of the change that she made?"

"Yes, she and the doctor discussed it, and he agreed."

"Well...I would simply like to hear from the doctor himself, if that's all right," said Ted. "We had a very positive appointment with the doctor, and in fact he's the one who suggested the increased amount, not me. I just want to clarify that he ordered this."

"The doctor is much too busy with other patients," she said.

"I'll be happy to wait," Ted said. "Could you please just have him pop in quickly to confirm the increased dosage?"

"You're already taking quite a lot of medication," she remarked.

I was appalled at her scolding attitude. The door was open and the nurse had stepped into the hallway at that point--this was a clear HIPAA privacy violation.

A different nurse entered the room after several minutes, stating that everything was "all set."

"What exactly is all set?" Ted inquired. "And what about the changed course of treatment?"

"The course of treatment will stand as dictated by the P.A.," said this nurse. "She sent a text message to the physician and that was the decision."

"Something's not right here," Ted said, "I was originally told they discussed it in person. Now you're telling me that the P.A. messaged the doctor. I just need to speak with the doctor directly about this."

The nurse refused, so Ted requested another appointment with the doctor.

"You can't have an appointment until July."

"This is not acceptable--" Ted started.

"You can communicate with us via the electronic Patient Portal," the nurse interjected.

"I've encountered many problems with it in the past. I would much rather speak with someone in person," Ted said.

"You can phone the office later and leave a voicemail."

"I will, but I will also be writing a letter to my doctor."

"Do not write a letter. Any letter you write will be intercepted."————————————————

We were taken aback by the turn of events. Ted phoned back later to leave his message for the doctor, but ended up speaking with the clinic coordinator, who repeated the denial of allowing Ted to speak with the doctor. Ted told this person also that he would be writing a letter to the doctor,

Ben Dales and B. B. Beaudreaux

only to be told any such letter would be intercepted and would not reach the doctor.

The next day, the clinic coordinator called Ted at home to state that Ted was being discharged as a patient of their pain clinic and of the doctor. He was told not to attempt to contact anyone there including the doctor, and that any attempt to do so would be intercepted before reaching the doctor.

The reason given for the discharge was "a breakdown of our provider/patient relationship."

The reason given for the discharge was "a breakdown of our provider/patient relationship." This is true, even if it does not acknowledge the cause of this "breakdown." The truth is the pain clinic's staff members deliberately prevented communication from the doctor to his patient, and additionally prevented communication from the patient to his doctor.

The underlying truth is that the P.A. prevented the dictated course of treatment by the physician (made during the one-time-per-year appointment with him) and had staff members acting on her behalf--not on behalf of the actual doctor or the patients. This physician assistant was not only making medical decisions instead of the physician, but she was changing the physician's directed course of treatment without explanation.

From the very first appointment with this P.A. and her staff nurses, it was a verbal struggle to make her (and them) understand the constant chronic pain Ted was experiencing and hence his needed course of treatment. It was almost as if he was being treated as someone "just out to get drugs" and not as a bona fide patient with unrelenting pain. This is further evidenced by the "Wean Schedule" included on the discharge letter, which demonstrates, incredibly, an opinion that Ted is able to survive without any pain medication at all. This last point illustrates discrimination against Ted due to his disability.

The above episode admittedly illustrates to what extent the events of the discharge blind-sided and consequently upset us. Complaints and grievances were filed with the corporate headquarters of the pain management company itself, with our insurance carrier, and with Medicare. Even so, nothing concerning the dis-charge decision ever changed. Later, as we were sharing the story of our discharge with others in our community, we learned of various incidents experienced by other patients of this P.A. and this clinic, which led to similar discharges of those patients as well.

In the weeks following the discharge in March, we went back to our primary physician (in the

Ben Dales and B. B. Beaudreaux

same city as the pain clinic and the one who had initially referred us to this pain clinic) to explain what had happened. He told us he was aware of others who were also discharged from that clinic's practice, and agreed to help us find another pain management clinic. A few days later, he gave us a list of four pain management offices of separate companies and a written referral from him for each one.

It was no short process to try to get into one of these clinics. First we started by trying to learn something about the clinics themselves before we began contacting them. As a result, we prioritized our list from top to bottom based on what we had learned. We contacted the first one, explained our need and our doctor's referral, and were advised they would review it and let us know. After a few days, we received a rejection. We continued on to the second one, experiencing pretty much the same process and then the same end result. The third and the fourth also rejected us.

It was easy to see what was going on. We were being blackballed by the previous pain management company that discharged us. With no other recourse, we were forced to return to our previous pain management doctor in Chicago, some three hours away, where Ted had gone prior to moving to Michigan. This was workable but certainly inconvenient, especially for him being forced to travel by car for six-plus hours round-trip in his chronic pain condition (given that he cannot sit upright for any length of time).

This continued as such for some four months until it was time for Ted's biannual appointment with his primary physician--the same one who had given us the four referrals. This appointment included a discussion of what had transpired with his search for a local pain management doctor and his new situation of being forced to return to Chicago every month. This doctor was empathetic, but offered no further solution. However, he did suggest that Ted speak with the office's Patient Advocate to see if she might be able to assist.

As it turned out, not only was the Patient Advocate a good listener in learning what had happened and in assessing Ted's needs, she came up with a few more suggestions of doctors who might be able to help him. This led to his having an appointment the next month with a doctor who agreed to see him--Dr. Mendelman. Although this doctor's location was over an hour away, it was still drastically closer than driving to and from Chicago.

Our very first appointment exceeded our expectations, both in a good way and in a not-so-

Ben Dales and B. B. Beaudreaux

good way. It was clear from the get-go that this doctor was ready to listen, ready to devote whatever time was needed to listen, and ready to understand rather than judge. Already this was many levels above the quality of service and treatment received at the previous clinic that discharged Ted. This doctor was also willing to meet with Ted on a monthly basis instead of farming him out to meet with some assistant. This procedure continued as such, with each appointment continuing to build mutual trust and respect between patient and doctor--much more like it should be.

A year and a half after our first appointment, this doctor's practice was abruptly closed, which hit us like a brick wall. We simply could not believe it, but somehow at the same time wondered to ourselves whether things had just been going along too well and that something so good could not last forever...just our usual luck and par for the course!

Our only option became going back to our original Chicago doctors, even though it meant a six-hour round-trip journey each month.

CHAPTER 40

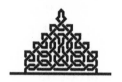

Ted: Life With Disability

After mistakes have been made by surgeons or other physicians, there are a myriad of reasons you do not get further help. The main one is because every time you come back to their respective offices, you remind them of the existence of that mistake. In addition, your presence is not really very good for their business, because in the waiting rooms people tend to talk to one another. Of course behind the closed doors of doctors' offices, the doctors and staff likewise talk. Though it would never be admitted, you have to wonder whether they are trying to find ways of getting rid of you.

Truthfully, they have to be really hoping you will move away or secretly hoping you die (cruel thought, but one very possibly true). Another option is that they wish that you will go elsewhere to another practitioner, even to the extent of

Ben Dales and B. B. Beaudreaux

dismissing you as a patient. And because they really do not want you going to some other practice right in the area, they can and will covertly "blackball" you, as I experienced.

The masses of scar tissue within my body led to a medical diagnosis of Intracranial Hypotension, a condition in which spinal fluid backs up in one's brain. I have accordingly come to expect that the more physical distress I experience, the more pain I experience. Whenever my pain medication wears off, more internal pressure builds up in my spinal column and brain. Another way to explain what is happening within me is that whenever spinal fluid movement is impeded by masses of scar tissue, the resulting backup of spinal fluid in my brain causes everything already described above along with neurological trauma, discomfort, and extreme distress. This distress level is so severely high that at times my only recourse is just to lie down wherever I happen to be.

This is a very tenuous predicament in which to find myself, as people or friends will rush to me and want to phone for an ambulance. If my medication were not available, that is exactly what would happen. Explaining what is going on is not easy, sometimes not even possible. It simply adds stress upon this already-stressed human.

What I usually tell people when these pain episodes happen is just to get me my meds and allow me to lie down until they start to take effect. I cannot tell my reader here how many people have thought I was on the verge of death when these types of traumatic situations have occurred.

Nevertheless, in the case of when you do finally end up moving, finding another doctor to look after you after the mistake has been made is another story altogether. Who really wants to take care of someone else's "Frankenstein?"

My personal boyhood hometown doctor in rural Wisconsin was Dr. Holcomb Everett. This gentle man, and truly a gentleman as well, was just such a caring doctor. The few times I had seen him as a child and young adult were mainly due to mundane maladies such as a cold or sore throat. When I came back to him years later in my late 30s with all the tragic stories about what had happened to me in the city, with great insurance that would pay for anything, he was really aghast.

Dr. Everett told me that having the "best" insurance in the world was not always the best thing for one's health--and that I was living proof of the fact.

"Would you have used the bone growth stimulator for the fusion instead of your own bone

Ben Dales and B. B. Beaudreaux

if you had not had insurance that would finance the device?" He asked.

"Well, probably not," I answered.

"And do you think you would have received the implant of their device if you had not had the absolute best insurance in the world to pay for it?"

I now realize just how correct Dr. Everett was.

Remember that bill I received for $103,000 following the surgical implant of the mini-neurostimulator, the one that caused the infection from which I nearly died (not to mention that upon seeing the bill, I again nearly died from shock)? Had I not kept and filed the letter of approval received prior to my surgery, I would have been on the hook for that amount. Dr. Everett knew it was a way for big corporate physicians and hospitals to make lots of money.

In fact, he shared privately with me that he had tried to retire early for just this reason. However, he soon came out of retirement for a while longer, because so many of his loyal patients relied upon him. As the years went on I began to realize that the things I went through were all due to greed and profit for those in the health field. My health was never a genuine concern for so many physicians, except for a select few such as Dr. Everett, Dr. Lottens, Dr. Allen, and Dr. Mendelman.

This was money that was being supplied by the medical device manufacturing industry to push the devices upon unsuspecting patients in pain who had good insurance. All they (that is, the corporate physicians' groups and pain management partnerships) needed was the proper diagnostic codes and the corresponding procedural billing codes that would open the doors to millions of dollars in fees and bonuses. This would also open up doors to the speaking fees that high-level surgeons could and would make by speaking at conferences promoted by the device manufacturers themselves. It was all such a big scam, but one by which, if again, you knew the proper diagnostic and procedure codes, would make millions for these doctors and hospitals and medical manufacturing companies.

The name of the billing and coding fiasco truly is the million dollar coding game, and it actually needs to be labeled as fiction to be believable. To quote the venerable Samuel Langhorne Clemens, memorable to us as Mark Twain, "Truth is stranger than fiction." In actuality, the complete quotation reads, "Truth is stranger than fiction, because Fiction is obliged to stick to possibilities; Truth isn't."

Ben Dales and B. B. Beaudreaux

CHAPTER 41

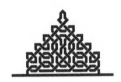

Deni: Life With Disability

Ted's agility was second to none. His quest for life experiences was exceeded only by his daring diligence. Never in my life had I such a close friend, now my spouse, who would attempt and succeed at just about anything and everything he decided to pursue.

I was amazed by his physical prowess. He could do flips off the low diving board into the pool. He could do multiple flips from the high one. The prowess flourished on land as well. He could walk on his hands. He could climb trees easily. He could do cartwheels and backflips. He could juggle. He excelled at most sports and games he tried.

Years ago, he mentioned he loved to play ping pong and asked if I wanted to play. I had observed his success in sports and I was a bit intimidated. However, I had grown up playing a lot of pool and ping pong at my grandparents' home at least every week if not more. I could always hold my own.

We decided to play a game of ping pong. It was a close contest and I won. This literally thrilled me; I had just found something at which I could beat him. We played a second game with the same result. I was finally at long last feeling I had found something I could excel at over him. That's when Ted grinned.

"Hey, I'm going to switch back to my right hand, okay?"

Hearing this, my shocked excitement quickly dissolved into resignation. Yes, he was a "rightie" and had been losing to me using his left hand, a small but important detail that I had not noticed in my excitement of the games.

It was the same when we played pool. When I did manage to win a game over him, I always wondered how much of a fluke it really was. Often the only time I won was when Ted was careless enough to scratch with the eight-ball, an automatic loss of game.

It was not just in sports and games, though, when he excelled (although he has countless volleyball trophies and medals that show otherwise). He was able to plan and accomplish

Ben Dales and B. B. Beaudreaux

just about whatever else he wanted to. He did an entire "makeover" of a beat-up Oldsmobile Cutlass his aunt had owned and he proudly carted me around in it. He painted beautiful landscapes and portraits. He developed into a gourmet chef. He was a self-made musician, both vocally and instrumentally (the cello). He purchased and redid a historic Craftsman bungalow in the Beverly Hills neighborhood of Chicago. The barren double city lot upon which this home sat, he developed into an award-winning garden that the locals demanded be a part of the annual Beverly Hills Garden Walk for five consecutive years.

When time came for my retirement from teaching in Chicago's public schools and the accompanying requirement that all city employees must actually live within the city limits, we found an unfinished newer home across the lake in Michigan. Though it was a nice house with the right price (from foreclosure), we once again had our work cut out for us. Out of the three separate levels, the entire first level and part of the third level were unfinished. Of course this was custom-made for his wonderful planning skills to apply to our needed project.

Realizing most of what needed to be done was beyond our current abilities, with his being disabled and my being continually older (retirement age by now), we found locals to do what we could not. This was largely helped by the fact that our closest neighbors were lifelong local residents. They literally knew everyone, whom to trust and depend upon for good work and whom not to. Although it took some money and some doing, it mostly took time and patience so that we could follow his careful plans to make this unfinished house into a showplace for our retirement home.

I hoped that Ted would never lose his mindful abilities in planning ahead for just about everything, even if he no longer possessed the same in his physical abilities.

The End Continues

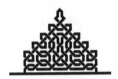

A voice. I hear…a voice.

I feel my hand being held. *Who's there? Have I arrived…?*

Oh, thank you God, for taking me home.

Who is holding my hand?

I have a hand…?

A soft voice is calling me. Very faintly, I hear my name. And again, and again.

Is this God?

Who is with me?

I hear my name again. I see light. *Have I made it to Heaven?*

The voice is familiar. Of course it is. How could it not be? I feel comfort and love.

I am seeing more light. A shadow appears.

My God, it looks like Fran. Fran is in Heaven with me?

I am disoriented but aware. I hear another voice, someone saying, "Can you hear me?"

Who would be asking me such a thing in Heaven?

I see a face. It is Franny for sure.

I hear another familiar voice, asking me if I can hear. It is Dr. Rand. *What is he doing here?*

"Am I gone?"

A calm voice answers, "You may be gone, but you're still on Earth."

"Dr. Rand? Franny? What is happening?"

"Ted, can you hear us?"

"Yes. I can hear you. And I can *see* you both. Where am I?"

"My dear one, you were hysterical," Dr. Rand said. "I had to sedate you."

"But why am I still here?" I asked.

"You started convulsing," Franny explained.

"I had to sedate you, knock you out," Dr. Rand repeated. "I was afraid you were going to have a stroke. We couldn't understand what you wanted."

"Franny? Am I still alive?"

"Of course you are."

"You were incoherent and as I told you, I cannot make this decision for you," Dr. Rand said. "You have to be a stable frame of mind to make the decision to end your life, and you simply were not in that frame of mind. I had no other choice but to calm you down until we could talk this over again."

I looked at my arm. There was no IV. There was no catheter.

"But...I said to do it, didn't I?"

"Yes. You did, but again, you were in no way capable of making that decision," Dr. Rand said. "I will come back tomorrow. I think we need to look at another way to treat your pain. One that does not mean ending your life--at least not at this time."

"But, I don't feel the pain!"

"Well," he chuckled, "that's because it took a lot of medication to put you out. We can treat you here with other medications that could give you hope and bridge the gap until a solution is discovered to control your pain. In any event, right now, I know you are not ready to say goodbye."

"Franny, will you stay here with me?" I asked.

"Of course I will. I am here for you. We are here to help you, not hurt you. You still have too much life left in you to end it now."

"I'll be back tomorrow," said Dr. Rand, glancing at Franny, "but I know that our friend here has a great many more things to accomplish in his lifetime."

"Just relax, my dear," Franny said to me. "You need to rest for now." She and Dr. Rand both rose and walked toward the door to the foyer, speaking in French.

I was still trying to understand what had just happened. I was relieved that they were not going to allow me to exit.

Fran came back to the familiar blue sofa and sat with me. I tried to focus on the large window with the paper-like blinds.

"Ted, you're not ready for this, not now."

"But what will I do?" I asked. The future seemed uncertain. I was nervous at the thought of facing the pain once again.

Ben Dales and B. B. Beaudreaux

"We will make sure you have the medical treatment to keep you comfortable and happy until you decide that it really is the right time," she said.

"But the pain will be back."

"No, we will give you anything you need to keep the pain at bay. You will live, for now. You have things to do. You need to tell people your story. You couldn't do that if you were leaving now, could you?"

"Well, no. But can I stand the pain?"

"Ted, we will make sure you are not suffering from pain. Please don't worry about that now. You need to rest. I'm going to make you some soup and then we'll talk some more."

I'm alive.

Fran was right. So was Dr. Rand. They knew I was not yet finished. I had to tell others what happened to me. I needed to tell my story. If I did so, maybe others in my condition would not need to suffer again and again as I have.

As I was traveling home from Belgium, I kept thinking about how Dr. Rand told me I wasn't ready. You have a story to tell.

Dr. Rand made it quite clear to me I had a story to tell. One which I had told dozens of physicians, only to have them brush me off as if it were nothing.

While still out of the country, I decided to call Deni. I couldn't help how gruff and disgusted I felt, although not because of anything that was said or told to me. It was not because of the questions about my "trip" that was thought to be a vacation. No, I was simply disgusted about returning to the country where I knew I would have to deal with all that same nonsense and greed that crippled me to the point I had been willing to euthanize myself just to stop the suffering.

Deni couldn't have been nicer to me on the phone. Somehow, through all the contempt I felt towards the very systems to which I was returning, I knew there would be at least one person to empathize with me--Deni. When I arrived back in the U.S., Deni was waiting for me with a smile and the usual questions one asks of someone who has taken a voyage.

"How was the trip?"

"Who did you meet?"

"What kinds of meals did you have?"

My answers were bland and curt. I think Deni thought I was just tired, or rather, exhausted, because I had been traveling alone "without assistance."

The drive back home was spent more in silence than anything. My thoughts drifted from the Belgium trip to the pets I'd had during all that transpired. With both of my dogs toward the end of their lives, I had made arrangements in advance for my local vet, Dr. Shawl, to come by the house to end their lives if it would not come to pass naturally. Heidi and Algonquin both had the grace to stop eating, find their appointed comfortable spots by the fireplace, and slowly, although surely with difficulty, finally pass away.

This is exactly the opposite of what happened with my cat, Blueberry. She had developed cancer internally before I could detect it and by the time I did, it was too late. During her last weekend, I was tending to her as best I could while praying that she would just pass away peacefully. During that sleepless weekend, she kept on breathing through the pain and purring intermittently. Nevertheless, she just would not die naturally.

On Monday morning after that long weekend, I found myself crying at the animal hospital with Blue wrapped in a blanket in my arms while waiting for the doors to open for business. When Dr. Shawl saw me, her face filled with anguish.

"Ted, why didn't you call me? I would have come over immediately."

"I was just hoping she would die naturally."

After we took Blue into the exam room, Dr. Shawl took one look at her and said, "Oh, yes, my little darling. It's time to go."

Dr. Shawl struggled to find a vein in her arm and paw. "Her legs are so calcified from toxins that have built up in her body, I can't get to a vein. I'll have to inject her directly into the heart."

She came back to the exam room with a long syringe, eerily similar to the one Dr. Rand had pulled out just before I went unconscious in Belgium.

"Dr. Shawl," I stopped her. "I want to do this. Blueberry is my cat."

"I can't legally let you do this," said Dr. Shawl. "I would lose my license if anyone found out that I let you take care of this."

"Then you insert the needle, but don't inject the dose."

"But what will that do?"

"Please, please let me do this."

Ben Dales and B. B. Beaudreaux

She inserted the large needle straight into the heart of my precious fluffy friend who had been with me all those years. After the needle was inserted and her hand was still on the pump, I put my finger over her thumb and pushed her thumb down to empty the lethal dose into the heart of my little grey fur ball who had kept vigil by me every time I had been lying in bed recovering from the many surgeries that came to cripple me.

At that moment, I understood Dr. Rand's compassion for helping his patients transition from suffering.

Blueberry was buried in a beautiful field near a lake with majestic trees and wild flowers growing all around her. Shortly after she died, I kept finding small hearts everywhere I would go. I found paper hearts, little red plastic hearts, heart-shaped hair barrettes, puffed-up fiber hearts, heart swizzle sticks, a scarf with hearts as its design, a glittered red heart, a felt heart, a keychain heart that had been discarded by whomever had used it. I received a card from a friend in the mail which read, "My heart goes out to you at the loss of your pet." Someone left a rosary of small pink hearts in my choir robe. Exiting the car one day, the wind blew a red ribbon with hearts all over it straight at me. Someone even gave me a Valentine box of candied hearts.

It was all so uncanny and overwhelming. I found an old sheer purple jewelry bag where I could put all the hearts I had come across. I did not go looking for hearts nor did I buy any of them. These hearts just seemed to appear out of nowhere until slowly but steadily, the bag was filled over the winter.

The following spring, I planted a blueberry bush on the spot where Blue was buried. Not too long after, it bloomed with thousands of beautiful grey-white flowers, the exact color of my beloved little fur ball. In summer, the branches were weeping like a willow as they were overloaded with the largest blue-grey berries I had ever seen.

This is what occupied my thoughts during the silent parts of the ride back to our home. I thought to myself what a compassionate thing I had done for a little creature I had loved, and who loved me so very much. Why is ending the life of a suffering person so different from ending the lives of those so many people refer to as "members of their family" when their pets are alive and healthy?

As we pulled into the driveway and I slowly made my way out of the car, I wrapped my arms around Deni. I was holding back all the emotions that flooded my mind on the journey home. I held back, not because I was trying to stop the tears, but because I knew Deni would never truly understand or even believe why I had gone away in the first place. I did not want to hurt Deni.

It was on this ride back I decided I would never ever tell anyone, especially Deni, why I had gone on this trip and what my intentions were. That is, until I told my story here.

What changed my mind?

For too long, I kept silent. And so have many others who have been hurt by medical devices and practices. To keep silent is to bury all the stories. These stories need to be heard by people in positions of power--to bring light and recognition into our respective worlds of suffering. There are many people out there like me who do not get a second chance, and whose stories would not be told if they ended their suffering without letting others know what happened.

You too need to ensure that your suffering will not be in vain. You too need to share your story in some way or form or fashion. It is my hope that you will find the courage, the fortitude, and the will to follow through as I have, no matter how horribly you are suffering.

EPILOGUE: OUR LIFE TODAY

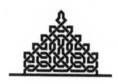

Ted: Enlightenment

Pain is exhausting. It squeezes the life out of a person.

All my passions for physical sports have been taken away, and I mean all of them. I cannot do any type of sport other than be in the swimming pool, and even that is getting difficult. Ever since the first surgery, I am unable to work. Deni and I ended up moving out in the country to an isolated house at the end of a lonely, half-mile, dead-end road. My home in the big city was just too much for me to handle. I have since had a lot of trouble finding a pain management physician in such a remote area, especially since the opioid epidemic ensued--even with my medical records, history, and photos of what happened.

My legs have atrophied. The tinnitus never went away either. It always seems the worst when all is quiet. Trying to get to sleep is next to impossible. The ringing never stops. It's like a constant siren going off in my head. If the pain is particularly bad, the tinnitus is correspondingly worse. Whenever I am in excruciating pain, the tinnitus is pulsatile--meaning it pounds in the brain with each heartbeat.

When I am unable to keep high levels of pain at bay with my medications, all the muscles in my body contract and make the normal flow of spinal fluid through my spinal cord and my brain even more difficult. This leads to what I can only describe as how one would feel if afflicted with the world's worst possible nausea after being exposed to the loudest ongoing city sounds imaginable. Think of feeling sick to your stomach and a bit dizzy while being in downtown Chicago and simultaneously hearing police sirens and fire truck sirens while standing beneath the elevated train tracks with a train passing over, and feeling the ground shaking beneath your feet. This is how I feel when the intracranial hypotension is putting pressure on my optic nerve. The pain is severe and constant.

Insurance battles have ensued because of blame on top of blame of who did what wrong. Pharmacies do not want to fill my prescriptions because of the actions of nefarious people who have abused the system to get their hands on "recreational" drugs. People of the world cannot comprehend that I have a disability when they look at me, even though I am unable to sit in an upright chair for longer than twenty minutes.

Of course I am irritable and cranky, but with all this going on, who wouldn't be?

However, with Dr. Rand's guidance, I was finally able to do things that I was only formerly able to do. I returned to swimming. I began anew with studying music. I hadn't been involved in music since I was a teenager and traveled down to Nashville to try to break into bluegrass and country music, but was unable to do so due to the financial need to work a "real job." I auditioned for a locally-renowned chorus and was asked to be a member, which I wholeheartedly accepted. This one act, being part of a musical group, was instrumental in my increased emotional well-being. It turned my attention from dwelling on everything that went wrong to what I was still able to do. Although singing was just a small part of who I was before, it made me feel needed once again.

It did not take long before I was trying out for solo parts in our two yearly concerts. I was able to share my music locally as well as regionally. Long ago I had dreams of making music a career and made friends with other vocalists and artists in the music industry in Nashville. Returning to the

Ben Dales and B. B. Beaudreaux

world of music reignited my old friendships with those who were still in the business of singing country and bluegrass music down South. Being able to pursue my passion for music again has been a saving grace in my life.

Am I angry? No, I have become enlightened. Now, I hope you are too.

Deni: Looking Back

Little did I realize I would take on the role of caregiver. Almost twenty-five years ago when we first became an item, if anything it was he who would likely one day assume that role...for me. After all, I am the one who is over sixteen years older than he. We used to joke about it, saying that someday he may be pushing me around in a wheelchair or at the very least helping me walk and get around. We have since learned the hard way that the likely future one foresees is never etched in stone. We can never predict with any level of accuracy.

And no, I am not saying that I now find myself pushing him around in a wheelchair. I am not helping him walk or get around, although I do most of the driving for him due to his inability to sit upright for given periods of time. I am a different type of caregiver. His afflictions are more hidden and less obvious to outsiders. His life has been changed forever by the unrelenting pain he is forced to endure. What he is now dealing with is something that profoundly affects my life as well.

I am not merely talking about helping him make special reservations at events and venues to accommodate the fact that he cannot sit in a normal seat or chair like everyone else. I am not merely talking about helping him cart around and carry his special chairs into these places. I am not merely talking about doing most of the driving to doctors and pharmacies and other sources of remedy (no matter how futile) so that he can somehow survive. I am not merely talking about doing the heavy-duty lifting and moving and all else that his disability does not allow him to do.

What I am talking about is being a caregiver who cares enough to listen to him as he tries to deal with what he is going through. I am the one who listens daily to his rants and ravings towards those who harmed him, knowing that he has every right to do so. I am the one who hears that he wishes there were a legal way to end it all. I also know I can do nothing to change what he is going through. Often when I try to say the right thing at the right time, it has just the opposite effect on him and upon his perception of me. It is at these times when my well-intended words seem to backfire on

Ben Dales and B. B. Beaudreaux

me and thrust me into the situation of enduring his verbal onslaught of words directed back at me.

I am a caregiver unable to give the care I really wish I could. I would just love, once or twice, to be able to remove the awful pain he is experiencing. I so much want to know the exact right words to say to help him and his demeanor instead of enrage him. I just want to be the caregiver who can truly help.

He still has big ideas and big plans for so many things he wants to accomplish or at least to see accomplished. At times I become frustrated, knowing I cannot do all the work it took two of us to accomplish before any of this happened. Doubly frustrating is the fact that I am unable to do all the work that I alone was able to do when we were first together, and before any of this happened.

Our life is so different now. We never know what each day will bring. I often watch him catching a quick nap in the late afternoon, exhausted by the pain and the constant ringing in his ears. The agile athlete has been replaced by a warrior who battles daily pain.

There are those who believe in the theory of "what goes around comes around." We may have a little faith in the validity of this theory as well. Perhaps it will give us some belated sense of relief and justice later on, who knows? In any case, it does nothing to help improve his condition and consequently to improve the journey we have been forced to tolerate.

The story of Ted and Deni lumbers on amidst all the daily trials and tribulations. It is alleged by forces from above that the hardest life challenges serve to make us stronger. Sometimes we wonder just how much more we can take and why us in the first place?

Since the day we first tied that legal knot all the way up to the present, we know our lives are much different than we'd ever suspected. We are different. We are grateful to have each other to turn to when needed, but we are also in each other's line of fire (and ire) when we become overwhelmed. We still somehow come back to the fact that we still have love for each other, no matter how disguised it may seem at times.

We use this to help each other get through the days and nights. Although we are unlikely to crochet or paint it on a wall hanging for our home, our mantra is summed up thusly:

Live through the challenges.

Laugh if and when able.

Love endures somehow.

Ben Dales and B. B. Beaudreaux

The Hippocratic Oath*

I swear by Apollo The Healer, by Asclepius, by Hygieia, by Panacea, and by all the Gods and Goddesses, making them my witnesses, that I will carry out, according to my ability and judgment, this oath and this indenture.

To hold my teacher in this art equal to my own parents; to make him partner in my livelihood; when he is in need of money to share mine with him; to consider his family as my own brothers, and to teach them this art, if they want to learn it, without fee or indenture; to impart precept, oral instruction, and all other instruction to my own sons, the sons of my teacher, and to indentured pupils who have taken the physician's oath, but to nobody else.

I will use treatment to help the sick according to my ability and judgment, but never with a view to injury and wrong-doing. Neither will I administer a poison to anybody when asked to do so, nor will I suggest such a course. Similarly I will not give to a woman a pessary to cause abortion. But I will keep pure and holy both my life and my art. I will not use the knife, not even, verily, on sufferers from stone, but I will give place to such as are craftsmen therein.

Into whatsoever houses I enter, I will enter to help the sick, and I will abstain from all intentional wrong-doing and harm, especially from abusing the bodies of man or woman, bond or free. And whatsoever I shall see or hear in the course of my profession, as well as outside my profession in my intercourse with men, if it be what should not be published abroad, I will never divulge, holding such things to be holy secrets.

Now if I carry out this oath, and break it not, may I gain for ever reputation among all men

for my life and for my art; but if I transgress it and forswear myself, may the opposite befall me.

* The Hippocratic Oath is an oath historically taken by physicians. It is one of the most widely known of Greek medical texts. In its original form, it requires a new physician to swear, by a number of healing gods, to uphold specific ethical standards.

Ben Dales and B. B. Beaudreaux

CPSIA information can be obtained
at www.ICGtesting.com
Printed in the USA
LVHW111359101219
640051LV00001B/3/P